Ayurveda for the Childbearing Years

a primer

Terra Rafael

Ayurveda for the Childbearing Years

ISBN 978-0-557-14703-8

Dedicated to the One I love.

Blessings on my Ayurvedic teachers and their teachers –

Deepak Chopra, Sarasvati Buhrman, Alakananda Ma,

Dr. Vasant Lad, David Frawley,

John Douillard, Dr. Nita Desai, and Dr. Sarita Shrestha.

Foreword

I became drawn to Ayurveda when I was a busy home-birth midwife, supporting women in pregnancy, birth, and postpartum with natural means. Why did some herbs and therapies work for one person with a condition, while another person with the same condition didn't respond favorably to that same help? I saw that a piecemeal approach to using natural remedies was based on symptomatic treatment—which is one of the problems with western medicine.

A holistic approach deals with the person more than with the disease, encouraging and supporting the natural healing responses in that person. While in Phoenix at a midwifery meeting, I heard a tape by Deepak Chopra, someone influential in popularizing Ayurveda in the US. Chopra's charismatic address led me to look further into Ayurveda. The principles and applications fit my own intuition and experience in my body. From there I began my studies in earnest.

That was over a decade ago. After hours & hours of classes, reading and practicing, Ayurveda delivers all & more than what it promised me. It is both as simple & commonplace as the sun rising each day, and as complex as all of the forces that allow that to happen & us to view it. What I'll explain to you here is for simple & commonplace use. To delve into the more complex levels takes time & dedication. And I encourage you to go for that level, if you, like me, feel that pull to integrate your knowledge with this rich system.

Table of Contents

Primer on Ayurveda

What is Ayurveda & how is it useful?

Ayurveda is the 5,000 year old system of healing from India which teaches "the way of life". This way does not dictate one path for all, but offers understanding about the basic energies of the universe and how they manifest in differing amounts in each person. Maintaining one's own personal balance of energies amid the changes of life allows mind, body & soul to express in the healthiest possible way. Ayurveda is being talked about more & more in alternative health magazines and yoga communities. It is a sister science of yoga.

Ayurveda, like midwifery, finds intuition to be the highest authority. Sometimes people get bound up in the guidelines about how to balance through diet, lifestyle, and therapies, making them into rules written in stone, and then get discouraged when they can't follow them exactly, right from the start, so they quit. This perfectionistic view is a disease in itself. Just as written protocols might guide a new practitioner or lend support when we are too tired or out of balance, so too the guidelines of Ayurveda. They help us get to the point where we are clear enough & experienced enough to 'go with the flow' with confidence. Ayurveda even recommends methods to increase our native intelligence, increasing our mental clarity.

The Doshas, Constitution, and Current Condition

The aspect of Ayurveda that is most commonly known is the DOSHAS. "Dosha" means that which can go wrong. These are basic energies that act within all living beings. VATA comes from ether and air elements. PITTA originates from fire and some water. And KAPHA comes from water & earth elements. The qualities of the three doshas are outlined in Table A, below. All of us have all three of the doshas operating within us. We need all of the qualities working at doing different jobs in our bodies.

Each individual is born with a set capacity to hold each of the doshas in their system. This is called the CONSTITUTION. Our constitution is created by three main influences: the environment at conception (especially the condition of the parents); the prenatal environment; and spiritual influences. We determine the constitution through investigation of long term trends of the body & mind, and by pulse diagnosis. The constitution is the benchmark of health. Constitution is expressed as ex. Vx Py Kz, with x, y, and z a numbers from 1 to 3, according to the proportions of the particular constitution. Examples are: V3P2K2, V1P3K3, V2P2K3, V3P1K2, etc.

Our current CONDITION shows if we are filling or exceeding our capacity for the doshas in our body/mind system. It is influenced by what we eat, the weather, the emotions of people around us, our activities, our daily routine(or lack thereof), how we breathe, our own thoughts & emotions and so forth. Maintaining a relatively stable condition requires adjusting our choices to balance out influences which are beyond our control, such as change of the seasons or uncontrollable events in our lives. The condition is expressed as Vx Py Kz, same as the constitution, making it easy to compare the two. The levels of the condition might go as high as 4.

When current condition levels match constitutional levels, then our system is balanced & expresses optimally. But this balancing act is more like surfing a wave than a static balance. The more you can tune into a developing excess and learn what adjusts the levels, the better you ride those waves.

The condition is determined by noticing changes in our body/mind, and by pulse diagnosis. The advantage of pulse diagnosis is that subtle changes show up in the pulse before manifesting on the physical level and can be addressed more gently before they become physical.

Dosha	Vata	Pitta	Kapha
Elements	Space & Air	Fire & Water	Water & Earth
Main Qualities	Dry, Cold, Light, Changeable, Mobile, Rough	Hot, Sharp, Oily, Spreading	Moist, Cold, Heavy, Viscous, Inert, Dense
Main Seat	Abdominal/ Pelvic area	Solar plexus	Chest
Balanced Expression	Flowing & Flexible, Enthusiastic, Creative	Focus, Intelligence, Good digestion & assimilation, Leadership	Strength, Endurance, Steadiness, Structure
Excess Expression	Constipation, shakiness, gas, cramps, fatigue, overwhelmed, fearfulness, distracted	Heartburn, skin conditions, diarrhea, inflammation, anger, irritability, overly critical	Excess weight, excess mucous, congestion, lethargy, denial, greed
Primary Body Tissue & Functions	Bones, nervous function, breathing, elimination, hearing	Red blood cells, skin, muscles, digestion, vision	Kidneys, plasma, fat tissue, cerebrospinal fluid, taste, fluid balance,

Table A : The Doshas in the Body

The Subdoshas

Each dosha has five SUBDOSHAS which operate more specifically. Especially of note for childbearing is the apana vayu, which rules the movement of menses, & childbirth.

Subdoshas are examined through questioning and pulse diagnosis.

SUBDOSHAS	LOCATION	DIRECTION	FUNCTION
VATA-VAYUS			
Prana	senses, brain, throat, chest	inward	taking in
Udana	chest, throat	upward	putting out ie exhaling
Samana	small intestine	balancing	absorption
Vyana	heart outward to whole body; especially extremities	outward	circulation
Apana	pelvis	downward	regulate pelvic holding in & letting go
PITTA			
Sadhaka	brain and heart	inward	inner fire
Alochaka	eyes	upward	receive light
Pachaka	stomach, liver/spleen	equalizing	digestion, discrimination
Bhrajaka	stomach	outward	digestion warmth & sunlight
Ranjaka	liver	downward	warmth in blood
KAPHA			
Tarpaka	brain, heart, nerves	inward	calmness, stability, happiness
Bodhaka	tongue, sensory in head	upward	taste, knowledge, perception
Kledaka	stomach-alkaline & mucous lining	balancing	liquifies food
Sleshaka	joints, limbs, skin	outward	cohesion & ease of movement
Avalambaka	chest, heart & lungs	downward	lubrication

Table B, Subdoshas

Another important concept is the TISSUES. In Ayurveda seven tissue levels are recognized.

Dhatu or Tissue	Dosha & elements	Subtissue	Waste Products
Rasa or plasma	Kapha Water	Breast milk or menstrual blood	Kapha dosha / phlegm
Rakta or blood	Pitta Fire & Water	Blood vessels & tendons	Pitta dosha / bile
Mamsa or muscle	Kapha Earth/water & fire	Ligaments & skin	Earwax, naval jelly & toe jam
Medha or fat	Kapha water	Omentum	Sweat
Asthi or bone	Vata Earth & air	Teeth	Nails & hair
Majja or marrow/nerves	Kapha water & earth	Sclerotic fluid of eye	Tears & eye secretions
Shukra/Artava or male/female reproductive	Kapha water	Ojas	Smegma

Table C, Tissues of the Body

Each tissue level feeds the next tissue level, going from the densest to the most subtle. We begin with the digested food, which feeds the plasma. The next level, blood, is fed by some of the plasma being digested into it. Then blood feeds muscle and so on. This means that, in general, to nourish the reproductive level all of the other tissues must have been nourished and digested well so that the next level can receive nourishment. It also takes about 7 days for the nutrition to move from one level to the next--- thus about 47 days to build the reproductive tissue. Tissue health can be ascertained by examination & questioning and by pulse diagnosis. In addition to foods, special herbs can be used to build tissues or increase digestion of that tissue level.

Agni or Digestive Fire and Ama or Digestive Toxins

One more key concept in Ayurveda is the relationship between AGNI or digestive fire and AMA or digestive toxins. When digestion is strong, the digestive toxins in the body are diminished. This is important, since most diseases have ama as a component. It's also true that when there is a lot of ama, digestion is impeded. Thus a cycle can be set up: digestion being off leads to ama which further reduces digestion and creates more ama. Maintaining healthy digestion is primary.

Ayurveda determines ama through questioning, tongue diagnosis, and pulse. Ama can be reduced and digestion increased by lifestyle & eating habit changes and by herbs. Especially effective is the cleansing & rejuvenation process of Pancha Karma (which isn't suitable during pregnancy or breastfeeding but excellent preconception and post-

post-breastfeeding). Pancha Karma expels ama out of the body, rekindles agni and then feeds the body tissues with rejuvenative herbs. See the Chapter "Caring for Digestion" for more details about helping digestion.

Basic Ayurvedic Self Assessment

•Basic Pulse Check for Vata, Pitta and Kapha –
Reach around from behind the wrist so the pointer finger is closest to the hand. Place the first three fingers on the thumb side of the wrist, under the bone prominence below wrist lines. Press gently until you feel a pulse.

What is the quality of the pulse under each finger?
- Vata quality is wiggly, like a snake
- Pitta quality is jumpy, like a frog
- Kapha quality presses with fullness and grace, like a swan swimming.

Which finger is dominant?
•Home of the Vata pulse is under your index finger
•Home of the Pitta pulse is under your middle finger
•Home of the Kapha pulse is under your ring finger

•Observe your stools – Healthy stools according to Ayurveda are light brown, the consistency of ripe bananas, and float;
•Vata tendencies in the stool make it   darker or harder;
•Pitta tendencies make it lighter colored and more loose;
•Kapha tendencies make large amounts, tinged with mucous;
•Ama or toxic tendencies include undigested food, sticky (need lots of toilet paper), and sinking.

•Observe your tongue – Use natural light to see by if possible. If there's more than a very thin coat that means there's some ama or toxins. Look for daily change— when there's more it indicates digestive changes or foods you ate yesterday don't digest well for you now.

Location gives more clues.
- Back of tongue=colon toxins (Vata seat) ;
- Middle=small intestine toxins (Pitta seat)
- Front= stomach (Kapha seat).

Color?
- Thick white=Kapha toxins;
- Greasy yellow=Pitta toxins;
- Brownish, grayish, blackish = Vata toxins.

Other features?
- Red dots or areas of tongue = Pitta
- Cracks; tooth indentations around edge; tremors = Vata
- Frothiness = Kapha

•Observe your energy level – high or low? Does it change at different times of day?

•Note any pain or tenderness in the body – always in same spot? Where?
- o Upper back, neck, stomach, chest = Kapha
- o Mid back, liver, gallbladder, solar plexus, small intestine = Pitta
- o Lower back, pelvis, colon, thighs = Vata

•Note your appetite – steady?
- o Fluctuate =Vata ;
- o always hungry=Pitta ;
- o Never hungry? Kapha dullness or ama

•Observe the taste in your mouth when you wake up-
- o Bitter, Astringent, Dry = Vata
- o Sour = Pitta
- o Sweet, salty, thick saliva = Kapha

After determining if there is imbalance or toxins you can eat and treat yourself accordingly. For acute toxins-skip breakfast and drink ginger tea instead-

Vata -- skip breakfast only,

Pitta and Kapha -- wait for appetite to return before eating.

When you find a dosha out of balance, follow diet and lifestyle balancing to keep it from overflowing. If you are confused by what you see, if it seems like you frequently have more than one dosha out of balance, or you have serious problems, be sure to go to an Ayurvedic Practitioner. See the Resources and Reading List Chapter for help finding an Ayurvedic Practitioner, if you need one.

Thanks to Alakananda Ma for sharing much of this teaching. She can be reached at Alandi Ayurvedic Gurukula, in the Resources & Reading Lists chapter.

Balancing with Food

Qualities of the Doshas and Food

Vata -   Vata is dry, light, expansive, rough, cold, changeable, subtle, and quick. When you have an excess of these qualities you must help balance them with their opposites & avoid adding more of them.
•   Get the tastes that balance Vata- predominately sweet, sour, & salty. Eat heavy, moist, soupy,& warm cooked food with digestive spices added.
•   Avoid cold foods or beverage, and stimulants like caffeine, alcohol. (a little beer or wine w/ meal OK occasionally) Avoid junk food & microwaved food. Avoid nightshades-potatoes, tomatoes, eggplant, bell peppers.

Pitta -   Pitta is hot, oily, sharp, moist, fluid, and sour. Avoiding these qualities and using their opposites will help to balance an excess of Pitta.
•   Get the tastes that reduce Pitta - mainly sweet, bitter & astringent, with fresh, raw foods & juices.
•   Avoid alcohol, chilies, tomatoes & other acidic foods, tea, coffee, & fried foods. Avoid nightshades.

Kapha - Kapha is heavy, cold, moist, stable, sweet, soft, sticky, dull, smooth. Again, using opposites and avoiding these qualities will help balance an excess of Kapha.
•   Get the tastes that reduce Kapha - pungent, bitter & astringent, including warm, light, & dry foods with spices.
•   Occasional fasting or skipping a meal is good.
•   Avoid cold foods or drinks & sweet, heavy, or rich foods..

Qualities of the Six Tastes

Sweet
- Qualities:Cooling, Wet, Heavy;   Gives Grounding: Made up of Earth & Water elements
- Balances Vata & Pitta, Increases Kapha.
- Use turbinado sugar, sucanat, gur, jaggary, maple syrup; GRAINS are the best sweet food to use freely (unless you have a sensitivity to them).
- Excess leads to Kapha excess: obesity, flaccidity, heaviness, weak digestion

Sour
- Qualities:: Heating, Wet, Light. Improves digestive fire & adds bulk. Made up of Earth, & Fire elements.
- Balances Vata , increases Pitta & Kapha.
- Use lime, apple cider vinegar
- Too much makes teeth sensitive, thirstiness, blinking eyes, goose bumps, liquefies Kapha, aggravates Pitta, causes toxins to build in the blood, wastes muscles, creates sores & wounds to suppurate, burns stomach, chest & heart.

Salt
- Qualities: Heating, Wet, Heavy. Increases digestion, moistening. Made of Water & Fire elements
- Balances Vata – in moderation: the most restricted of the taste for all doshas, increases Pitta & Kapha
- Use real salt/ rock salt, which has minerals still in it. Sea salt only if unrefined & yellowish. Salt shouldn't be pure white or it has had minerals removed & is less healthy.
- By itself or too much increases Pitta, stagnates the blood, makes thirst, fainting, burning, muscles wasting & aggravates skin conditions. It can cause malignant tumors to break apart & spread. Causes wrinkling of skin &

falling of hair, loss of virility & teeth, and obstructs the senses.

Pungent

- Qualities: Heating, drying, light. Increases digestion. Made of Air & Fire elements.
- Balances Kapha, increases Vata & Pitta.
- Examples: cayenne, peppers, salsa
- Too much weakens virility, creates delusion, weariness, dizziness,& burning; reduces strength, increases thirst, tremors, piercing & stabbing pains.

Bitter

- Qualities: Cooling, drying. Restores taste & detoxifying. Made of Air
- Balances Pitta & Kapha, increases Vata.
- Examples Neem, greens
- Too much increases Vata, wastes tissues, causes roughness, emaciation & weariness.

Astringent

- Qualities: Dry & Airy. Earth & Air elements.
- Reduces Pitta, increases Vata & Kapha
- Examples yarrow, motherwort, choke cherries, some greens
- Excess drying of mouth, constipating, weakens voice, darkens skin, premature aging, retention of gas, urine, feces, and causes Vata diseases.

Caring for Digestion

- To rekindle the digestive fire: About 10 minutes before meals take Agni Kindler (see Recipe chapter) This will wake up your digestive enzymes naturally and get them into a rhythm. (Safe for pregnancy.)

- If you have absorption problems, immediately fol-low your meal with takram (see Recipe chapter)

- Drinking Cumin Coriander Fennel tea is another digestive help(in pregnancy, leave out the fennel). It burns body toxins, kindles digestion, and helps any gas move out. This tea helps your body self regulate its hormones and helps promote milk production postpartum as well! Mix equal parts of seeds. Use 1 tsp total of seeds per cup tea. Simmer 10 minutes, strain & drink.

- Try to eat at regular times. This habit allows your body to anticipate meal times by starting its digestive juices going at the usual time. It also reduces Vata.

- Eat your largest meal between 10 am and 2 pm when the digestive fire is normally at its peak.

- Don't overeat at a given meal. Overeating smothers the digestive fire, just as putting too much wood on a fire will eventually put it out. One guideline for how much to eat is to cup both of your hands in front of you. The amount you can hold in your hands is about how much your stomach can hold and do its job well.

- Eat food at room temperature or a little warmer. Eating with your fingers will make sure it is the right temperature. Test your tea with your little finger.

Digestive enzymes are temperature specific and evolved to work with room temperature food—not refrigerated , frozen or iced.

•	Allow 3 hours between solid food meals to allow digestion to be complete before new food is added to the system. Fruit digests faster when taken alone as a snack , so you can eat other food about 11/2 hours after fruit.

•	Don't drink much liquid with meals. ½ hour before or 2 hrs after. This avoids diluting your digestive juices, which would reduce their working capacity. Have soupy foods at meal time to avoid too much dryness instead of drinking. Or just sip a little warm water.

•	Chew food mindfully. The mouth is the first step of digestion—chewing well mixes the enzymes in saliva thoroughly with your food to begin the breakdown necessary for full digestion.

•	Use proper food combining as a rule. Occasional lapses may not be problematical, but daily or regular lapses will lead to serious toxic build up & the possibility of serious disease in the long run.
•	Avoid foods you know you don't digest well.
•	No fruits eaten with other types of foods
•	Melons always eaten alone

•	Milk always taken alone except for totally sweet fruit (ie. Dates, mangoes, figs) or cooked with basmati rice
•	Don't mix milk with dal, fish, or meat.
•	Don't take yogurt in a meal with meat.

•	Relax to allow for proper digestion. Talking lots, reading and other "head" activities can confuse your prana or life energy flow as to which way to flow and are bad for digestion. Avoid jumping up & down from the table or watching tv. Avoid emotionally upsetting topics & topics you don't want to take deeply into your body. Saying a prayer or sitting quietly for a minute or two before eating will allow you to slow down and let energy & blood go to digestive tract.

• Subtle qualities of food can become more important in the sensitive postpartum period. Fresh foods bring vital energy —avoid leftovers longer than 24 hours old. A pleasant atmosphere & appearance of food will make for better digestion—you'll feel more like taking it in.

• Don't eat & then sleep, exercise (except for gentle walking), or meditate—leave 2 hrs between them. Digestion works better in an awake state.

• Avoid exciting, stressful, or scary activities— when adrenaline is flowing, digestion is turned off to make more energy for fight or flight. Taking some deep, relaxing breaths or pray before meals to turn off the adrenals and avoid this problem.

• Follow the diet appropriate for your constitu- tion &/or current condition, as well as the season. For most postpartum women a Vata reducing diet is appropriate. (see suggested Vata diet modified for postpartum women)

Daily Balancing for the Doshas

Vata -   Vata is dry, light, expansive, rough, cold, changeable, subtle, and quick. Too much of these qualities in someone's life can imbalance their Vata. Governing motion, Vata rules neurological communications, movement of food through the digestive system, urinary control, sexual ejaculation, menstruation & childbirth. Its "seat", or place in the body where it is more predominant, is the colon/pelvic area. Fall & early winter are Vata times of year. Elder years are Vata time of life. 3 am- sunrise and 2-3 pm - sunset are Vata times of day. Vata is often more evident during pregnancy and especially postpartum. (If pregnant, always check to make sure any therapy you do is truly safe for pregnancy-everything suggested in this chapter is considered safe for pregnancy.) Vata can also be over stimulated by a lifestyle of irregular eating & sleeping, and quickly arising situations.

Balanced expression: The body is functioning smoothly; one feels life flowing. We feel alert, sensitive, enthusiastic, spontaneous, and creative.

Excess expression: The body suffers constipation, shakiness, cramps, gas, fatigue, or menstrual cramps before bleeding.   Emotionally, we feel overwhelmed, fearful, forgetful, distracted, moody, or sleep irregularly.

What to do if imbalanced in Vata? We warm, ground, contain, smooth, moisten, slow, steady.

- Have regular, moderate exercise, in moderate amounts, such as walking or hatha yoga
- Take warm, relaxing baths. Sip warm, vital water frequently through out the day. Listen to a stream or a fountain.

- Aromatherapy/incense - sandalwood, camphor, wintergreen, musk
- Use music to the calm, nurture, ground yourself. Avoid loud rock music or any loud noises.
- Calm your mind with gentle habits of reading, meditating, praying. Avoid fearful, worrisome or overwhelmed thinking. Avoid too much thinking or talking or studying. Avoid excess stimulation by media & computers.
- Be settled. Avoid moving homes, jobs, etc. too much. Do not travel too much, especially by airplane
- Have a routine- eat, sleep, BM at regular times soothes the body and mind.
- Slow, gentle self massage with sesame or almond oil, especially to feet, top of head, back, & abdomen or get massage from someone else regularly.
- Have time alone. Avoid overworking & too much socializing.
- Get regular sleep. Go to bed before 10 pm, earlier if possible. Get enough sleep.
- Get the tastes that balance Vata- predominately sweet, sour, & salty. Eat heavy, moist, & warm food with digestive spices added. Avoid cold foods or beverages and stimulants like caffeine, alcohol. (a little beer or wine w/ meal OK occasionally) Avoid junk food & microwaved food; avoid leftovers more than 12 hours old.
- Drink nourishing herbal infusions daily especially oat straw.
- Eat mindfully – Sit down while eating. Before eating sit quietly, breathe deeply, and give thanks. Chew thoroughly.
- Use color therapy - most colors good -pastel colors for sensitivity, avoiding lots of dark or heavy colors- or gems -emerald, jade, peridot set in gold; yellow sapphire, topaz & citrine & other yellow stones set in gold; ruby or garnet can help circulation & energy- & gem elixirs to work with the energy.

Pitta - Pitta is hot, oily, sharp, moist, fluid, and sour. Again, too much of qualities in a given individual will show up as a Pitta imbalance. Pitta governs digestion, assimilation & metabolism, on a tissue & cellular level as well as system level. Mental processing of experience is also ruled by pitta. Its seat in the body is the solar plexus, relating to liver, spleen & small intestine. Summer is the Pitta season; middle age the Pitta time of life; 10am-2pm and 10 pm -2 am the Pitta times of day.

Balanced expression: The body is taking things in well and using them properly. We are energetic, intelligent, confident, with right use of our will.

Excess expression: There is heartburn, cracking or itching skin, bad taste or odor from body, excessive thirst, diarrhea, inflammations, cramps with menstrual bleeding, or excessive heat in the body. We notice anger, irritability, unrestrained ambition, or criticism of ourselves or others.

What to do if imbalanced in Pitta? We want to cool, soften, calm, sweeten.

• Spend time out-of-doors in fresh, cool air, with cool lakes & streams, in gardens & flowers. Be careful not to overdo sunlight &/or heat or hot tubs. Bathe in moon light.
• Regular, cooling & calming exercise is best - guard against overdoing it & pushing yourself beyond 1/2 of capacity. Avoid too much competition.
• Take relaxing baths & showers, avoiding too hot of water. Drink vital, cool water. Listen to or wade in a stream or a fountain.
• Aromatherapy/incense-sandalwood, vetivert, henna, rose, lotus, jasmine, gardenia, honeysuckle, iris.

- Use music to calm & cool Pitta.
- Avoid dwelling on anger, jealousy, competition, being critical of others - stay with sweetness of speech, forgiveness, & contentment.
- Self inquiry is important in giving up tendencies to anger, overcritical or argumentative attitudes.
- Get moderate amounts of sleep, going to bed early (before 10 pm) & getting up early (before sunrise).
- Massage (with cooling coconut, sunflower, or ghee) - whole body or top of head, forehead, heart; by self or from another person.
- Get the tastes that reduce Pitta - mainly sweet, bitter & astringent, with fresh, raw foods & juices. Avoid alcohol, chilies, tea, coffee, & fried foods.
- Drink nourishing herbal infusions daily (esp. red raspberry, nettles, or red clover)
- Use color therapy - cooling white, blue or green; avoid very bright colors, esp. red; gray or brown is ok but avoid black- or gems -moonstone, clear quartz crystal, emerald, jade, peridot, blue sapphire, amethyst set in silver- & gem elixirs to work with the energy.

Kapha - Kapha is heavy, cold, moist, stable, sweet, soft, sticky, dull, smooth. Too much of these will result in a Kapha imbalance.Kapha governs the integrity & lubrication of the physical matrix of the body. Its seat is the chest. The wet, end of winter and the spring are Kapha time of year; childhood is Kapha time of life; and sunrise - 10 am and sunset - 10 pm are Kapha times of day.

Balanced expression: The body has great strength & endurance, fertility. We are steady, reliable, solid and dependable.

Excess expression: The body gains weight easily, loses with difficulty; excessive mucous, trouble with sugar metabolism, is congested or retaining fluids. We notice dullness, lethargy, denial, laziness, and heavy depression.

What to do if imbalanced in Kapha? We want to lighten, warm, clear,move & invigorate.

- Spend time out-of-doors in fresh air, in warm breezes. Sunbathe. Avoid coldness & damp.
- Get regular, daily, strong, aerobic exercise.
- Take invigorating, hot showers. Drinking moderate amount of warmed,vital water.
- Aromatherapy/incense -musk, camphor, cloves, cinnamon, cedar, frankincense, myrrh
- Use music to move the Kapha the energy; clearing & stimulating
- Following a discipline & enduring physical hardship are good for Kapha reducing. A detached mind is a useful quality to develop, avoiding greed, desire & sentimentality.
- Mental stimulation is important.
- Travel & pilgrimage is a useful form of Kapha reduction
- Less sleep helps reduce Kapha - staying up late may help. However, definitely avoid sleeping in the daytime.
- Any massage (dry or with stimulating oils like wintergreen, camphor, cinnamon) - whole body or foot/head/hands
- Get the tastes that reduce Kapha - pungent, bitter & astringent, including warm light & dry foods with spices. Occasional fasting or skipping a meal is good. Avoid cold foods or drinks.
- Drink stimulating herbal infusions of nettles and ginger tea.
- Use color therapy - warm & bright colors; avoid white, pink, or pale blue or green; some brown, gray,

& black- or gem therapy -ruby, garnet, cat's eye set in gold- & gem elixirs

By applying the simple & natural principles of Ayurveda for reducing excesses, we can not only help avoid deep seated diseases; we can also enjoy the creativity of balanced Vata, the energetic intelligence of Pitta, and the reliable steadiness of Kapha in ourselves & our families.

Sources & Further Reading :
Ayurvedic Home Remedies by Dr Vasant Lad
Ayurvedic Healing by Dr. David Frawley

Self Massage for Health

This is a is a firm, rhythmic, calming massage with a warm, specified oil to loosen toxins & excess doshas and begin to bring them into the digestive tract for elimination. The warm, oil massage is useful to balance Vata dosha and it is helpful for Vata people to do it at least three times a week. It's also useful before and after travel days to avoid formation of Vata excess. Kapha may benefit from dry brush massage and a more stimulating stroke.

- Oiling must be done on an empty stomach (at least 3 hrs after last meal), so for most people the morning is the best time.
- Warm the oil by putting a small plastic squeeze bottle of it in a sink or bowl of hot water for several minutes. If you are toxic by self assessment (heavily coated tongue) then use only castor oil for massage. Otherwise— sesame oil is best for Vata, sunflower oil for Pitta, and sesame for Kapha. There are also medicated oils for balancing the doshas available for the doshas from Banyan Herbs.
- Be sure to have old towels available to sit on and for under your feet (you will also need old towels for drying yourself after the showering or bathing.)
- Oil from head to foot, with most attention to head and feet, where there many marma energy points. Oiling & massaging them will help energetic balance of the organs. Continue at least ½ hour for a cleanse time; otherwise—do as much as you can.
  - o For the head- part your hair in several places and squeeze the oil directly onto scalp. The aim is to oil the head, not the hair. Then use open handed massage, more with the palms than the finger tips, in a circular motion.
  - o Up and down movement on the neck, long strokes along top of shoulders, then chest and breasts use

circular motion around the nipples. Up and down across solar plexus from one side all the way to the other.

    o   Clockwise, circular motion around umbilicus on abdomen

    o   Limbs—up and down motion on long parts, circular motion on joints (including shoulder and hip joints, elbows and knees)

    o   Feet- spend a good amount of time here—long strokes, pressing inward, circles on the sole of the foot

    o   Reach as much of your back as you can—include your lower back and buttocks

- Let the oil soak in 10 minutes while you prepare your bath, or go in the steam/sauna. Be sure not to become chilled at any point. You can wrap an old sheet around you or use a space heater if your bathroom is not warm enough.
- To remove excess oil from your scalp & hair, mix the shampoo with your oily hair BEFORE getting your hair wet. This will allow the shampoo to dissolve the oil more effectively. You may need to lather twice. (If the "messiness" of the oil in hair keeps you from the massage, try to at least massage the rest of the body with oil – some is better than none!)
- Be careful when oily not to slip in the tub and injure yourself. When you've completed your bathing, be sure to carefully clean the tub so no one will accidentally slip on the oily residue.
- Be sure to wash towels with plenty of soap & hot water to remove oil from them as much as possible. Recommended – use old towels that you don't mind throwing away when they get too oil/smelly.

Herbs for Women's Health and their Doshic Effects

Ayurvedic Herbs

Amalaki (amla) tonic, rejuvenative, alterative (use only pinch in pregnancy) PV-K+

Ashoka - prevent miscarriage, gyn problems, anti-toxic (constipates) P-VK+

Ashwagunda - tonic, rejuvenative, aphrodisiac, nervine   VK-P+

Bala - nutritive, rejuvenative – cool yet V-P-K-

Bamboo manna or Vamsa rochana - for too much dryness, emaciation, bleeding PV-K+

Brahmi - rejuvenative, blood purifier, fortifies immune system, good for kidneys VP-

Cardamon – digestant VK-P+

Castor oil- externally on hips for apana prana in labor or internally to purge to begin labor

Cumin/coriander/fennel tea- digestant (fennel not for early or fragile pregnancy)

Ghee - carrier substance for herbs, tonic to pitta, increases agni & ojas; V-PK neutral (don't mix in equal proportions with honey; not for high toxins, diarrhea, or parasites)

Guduchi -diuretic, liver tonic & stimulant P-

Licorice ghee – for perineal massage, also-cervical dysplasia (topical)

Lotus - nurturing tonic, aphrodisiac, astringent, nervine   PV-K+

Pippili – stimulant (use only small amount in pregnancy), digestant, expectorant, aphrodisiac VK-P+

Punanarva –(use with caution in pregnancy) diuretic, diaphoretic, laxative, rejuvenative   PK-V+

Shatavari - nutritive tonic, demulcent, digestive, rejuvenative, build milk PV-K+

Vidari - nutritive tonic, feeds tissues-good for placenta, demulcent, rejuvenative PV-K+

Western Herbs With Doshic Influences

Alfalfa leaf -digestion & vitamin K source PK-V+

Angelica - bring forth retained placenta VK-Po

Black cohosh- uterine toner for labor use in pregnancy PK-V+

Blue cohosh - stimulates contractions of uterus KV-P+

Chamomile - calcium, calming digestion PK-Vo

Cottonroot bark - Enhances oxytocin -helps stalled, ineffective labor & improves letdown reflex for breastfeeding V-KP+

Dandelion - liver toner PK-V+

Dong quai root - strengthen & balance uterus as tonic, nourish blood, mild liver stimulant, mild nervine; NOT during menses or pregnancy - may stimulate bleeding VK-Po

Echinacea - immune stimulant &lymphatic PK-V+

False unicorn root-femalehormone balancer/strengthenerthreatened miscarriage VK- P+

Ginger - for relieving nausea, increasing circulation, & digestion VK-P+

Licorice root - estrogenic, regulates hormonal balance, esp adrenal exhaustion - avoid if hypertension or water retention VP-K+

Lobelia - relaxant, balances out, causes vomiting & moderately toxic in excess K-PV+

Nettles - build blood, support kidneys & circulation PK-V+

Oatstraw - calcium & other nerve minerals, for stamina VP- K+

Passionflower - for calming & relaxing PK-V+

Pau d'arco - antifungal, alterative, antibiotic, anti-fever PK-V+

Peppermint - for gas, nausea & upset stomachs PK-Vo

Queen Anne's Lace /Wild Carrot - natural birth control, uterine stimulant KV-P+

Raspberry leaf - uterine tonic PK-V+

Red clover - nutritive, blood cleanser, hormone balancer PK-V+

Scullcap – calm nervous system, raise pain threshold PK-Vo

Shepherds Purse - Vit K & blood coagulation, vasoconstricting & mild uterine stimulant PK-V+

Spikenard - late pregnancy toner KV- P+

Squawvine - late pregnancy toner PK-V+

St Joanswort/ St Johnswort - for nerve pain PK-V+

Valerian - muscle relaxant VK-P=(inexcess)

Vitex or chasteberry - hormone balancer ???

Herbs to Avoid in Pregnancy

When in doubt - don't take it. Check with an experienced herbalist or Ayurvedic practitioner whenever possible before using any herbs in pregnancy, even if they seem to be totally unrelated to your uterus. Anything in excess should be avoided. Anything that imbalances your doshas should be avoided. Anything that stimulates menses (emmenagogues) or uterine contractions (oxytocics) should be avoided. Anything that is toxic should be avoided. Strongly hormonal herbs may throw off a normal balance - don't take them except in specially indicated situations. Antihistamines, laxatives & diuretics may also be dangerous during pregnancy.

If your pregnancy is in the first trimester or has shown any signs of fragility at any time in the pregnancy be more cautious = Fragile/Early (F/E). Some herbs may be ok if the pregnancy is firmly established -- that's why you may find different lists which include different herbs.

These lists are very comprehensive and conservative-you may use some, with knowledge & respect - but only if you take the risk & know enough about your body & the herb itself.

Ayurvedic Herbs to Avoid in Pregnancy

Aloe   **Berberis f/e or V**
All Bitter - scraping herbs
Fennel   **Fenugreek**
Ginger (a little   fresh OK)
Haritaki
Hing (a little in food OK)
Honey   **Jatamansi**
Licorice rt   Mahasudarshan
Neem   Nutmeg
Trikatu

Western Herbs to Avoid in Pregnancy

Antihistamines = Ma -huang, Ephedra, Osha
Laxatives = Flaxseeds, Aloes, Turkey Rhubarb, Cascara sagrada, Senna, Castor oil, Buckthorn
Diuretics = Buchu, Horsetail, Juniper Berries
Herbs Containing Steroid- like Factors =Agave, Ginseng, Licorice, Hops, Sage

Avoid these in the first trimester or if fragile pregnancy. Use sparingly later. =

Basil	**Caraway seeds**	**Celery seeds**
Ginger	**Fresh Horseradish**	
Marjoram	**Nutmeg**	**Parsley**
Rosemary	**Saffron**	**Sage**
Savory	**Tarragon**	**Thyme**
Watercress		

Goldenseal, which can irritate the uterus.

Emmenagogues - these can bring on menses through different actions; avoid =

**Angelica   Mugwort   Fresh Parsley leaves
Osha   Pennyroyal   Peruvian bk Rue
leaves Sumac berries   Saffron
Sweet flag rt   Tansy
Fresh wood sorrel
Fresh lemon balm   Bethroot
Birthwort   Black Cohosh   Blue Cohosh
Cottonroot Bark   European vervain
Ergot   Feverfew in flower   Ginger root
Hyssop leaves   Liferoot plant in flower
Lovage rt   Motherwort
Rosemary in flower
Marijuana female flowers
Mistletoe leaves**

Sources:
Dr. Vasant Lad -Notes from lecture on Ayurvedic Gynecology
Susun Weed, **Wisewoman Herbal for the Childbearing Year**
Drs. Vasant Lad & David Frawley, **The Yoga of Herbs** (to check doshic balance of herbs)
Rosemary Gladstar, **Herbal Healing for Women**
Peter Holmes, **The Energetics of Western Herbs Vol 1 & 2**

Menstrual Self Care

Menstruation - the monthly bleeding cycle of fertile women - is more than "the curse" or a "period". Ayurveda views menstruation as a cleansing time for a woman's body, which benefits it greatly. It is a time for self healing - if we arrange our lives to allow it to happen.

However, in this culture, women are expected to act "the same", no matter what, & our expected duties during the time of bleeding are no different than at any other time. Partly due to such lack of rest, care & awareness during the menses, many women in our culture experience menstrual problems and other related women's reproductive diseases, such as fibroids, endometriosis, infertility, or PID. By nurturing ourselves, maintaining energetic balance & avoiding build-up of toxins in the body throughout the cycle, women can find less discomfort and, in the long term, less disease.

Besides the cleansing action at the menstrual time there is another reason to take it easy at this time of the cycle. The uterus swells with fluids and becomes twice as heavy and larger in size in the few days before the bleeding begins. It also descends lower in the pelvic cavity. This stretches the ligaments that hold it in place. If there is a lot of bouncing, jarring or sudden twists or decelerations (as in a car accident) at this time the uterus is more susceptible to move out of her physiologic position, which can result in less blood flow to the ovaries and the uterus. If the circulation to the ovaries is impinged in any way it can garble communications between the pituitary and ovaries, which can confuse the cycle. And if the uterus is in an altered position it can lead to menstrual cramping and difficulties with conception. To remedy these problems Arvigo Techniques of Maya Abdominal Massage® is highly recommended. The protocol for ATMAM® includes teaching a woman a self massage technique to help maintain good blood flow and positioning between professional treatments. Rolfing & physical therapy can also help reposition the uterus.

By bringing awareness & care into the menstrual cycle, women also gain in experience that will serve them during a pregnancy. Excellent nutrition, maintaining energetic balance, taking nurturing herbs, getting adequate exercise & rest, relaxation practice – these promote both healthy menstrual cycles and healthy pregnancies. A woman who has been taught how to care for herself during her changing menstrual cycle is also practicing what she needs to know to take care of herself in pregnancy. She will have a healthier & more balanced start because by resting with her periods she will have honored the natural cleansing of menses, preserving reproductive health, both physically and energetically.

The emotional changes of the cycle prepare a woman for dealing with pregnancy. Women who take time to listen to themselves with awareness and care for themselves adequately find that heightened emotional sensitivity is not necessarily a call to bitchiness (although that too can be useful). It is also an opportunity to clarify what in their lives serves them & what does not. More alone time is a common need that women easily overlook at other times of their lives and often becomes more pressing during pre-bleeding & pre-birthing.

Women who have experienced the inward, downward pulling of energy during moon bleeding will be familiar with that feeling in its greatly intensified form during labor. Ayurveda calls this energy the apana vayu or apana prana. Healthy menstrual practices, as well as avoiding excessive holding back of the urge to urinate or defecate, help preserve the balance of this key energy for healthy pregnancy & birth.

Those who have experienced menstrual cramps can recognize the early labor sensation of the cervix beginning to open as a familiar one, not so scary. This brings the relaxed familiarity to early labor often considered possible only for those who have already given birth.

The Doshas & The Menstrual Cycle

During the menstrual cycle the energy of a woman may shift considerably. This is true more for some women than for others. By considering the possibility that we really aren't the same the whole month and acting & eating accordingly, imbalances may be avoided. Our women's bodies have their own seasons - just as Mother Earth does.

The cycle itself goes through the three different doshas:

Ovulation time until bleeding begins is Vata predominant. Apana vayu stimulates ovulation & helps the egg begin its journey down the fallopian tube. It rules degeneration of the endometrium. During the premenstrual phase, an out of balance apana vayu may push excess kapha, pitta or vata into uterus, creating different types of PMS - the woman's symptoms depend on the predominant dosha.

Vata imbalance creates overwhelm, worry, depression, and pre-bleeding menstrual cramps.

Pitta imbalance leads to irritation, anger, acne, and sore breasts.

Kapha imbalance creates lethargy, depression, and water retention.

Bleeding time is Pitta predominant.

Pitta imbalance leads to excessive bleeding & cramps during heavy bleeding.

Vata imbalance leads to clots and a slow cramping beginning to the menses.

Kapha imbalance leads to mucous in the menses.

Between bleeding time & ovulation is the Kapha predominant phase. The new endometrium is built, ojas (vital energy) is more predominant, love & compassion come more easily, she become more easily sexually aroused. Some Kapha women find this time is too Kapha for them, bringing lethargy, heaviness, or other Kapha type symptoms.

Ama & the Menstrual Cycle

Besides the effects of disordered doshas affecting the menstrual period, it may also be affected by excess ama or toxins built up in the body. The most common cause of ama is due to improper digestion. Another form is environmental toxins, many of which can negatively impact the reproductive systems of men and women.

In Ayurveda there are cleansing processes available called pancha karma to rid the body of built up toxins from incomplete digestion or other causes. Pancha karma can be undertaken with the help of a trained practitioner.

Cleansing herbs and healthy habits can also be used to increase digestive power and reduce ama from poor digestion. By ridding the body of these excesses, the menstrual time, which concerns purification of the woman's body, is not overloaded with its task and can work more easily.

The build up of ama can also be avoided by following simple dietary practices. See the Chapter on Caring for Digestion.

Self Care for Between Menses

*   Eat according to your constitution, following the ama reducing recommendations.

*   Exercise according to your constitution— neither over doing it (especially Vata or Pitta) or under exercising (more likely Kapha).

*   Get enough rest on a regular basis (Vata needs most, Kapha least).

*   Practice a daily form of turning inward - meditation, contemplation, chanting/singing/drumming, dancing, divination, prayer.

•   Always avoid holding back or forcing the urge to urinate or defecate as much as possible to protect apana vayu.

*   Use nourishing herbs (red raspberry, nettles, oatstraw) & food supplements (sea weed, bee pollen, etc.) that suit your constitution to support your nutrition. (The Yoga of Herbs by Frawley & Lad gives good information on this.)

•   Learn to do the Arvigo Techniques Maya Abdominal Massage® on yourself from a practitioner, or a Arvigo Techniques of Maya Abdominal Massage® Self Care class. This massage between moon times promotes health in the whole pelvic region, especially supporting the uterus & ovaries. Practice it regularly

Self Care for During Menses

*   Take time out for R-E-S-T. Some women ask their cycles to come on the weekends - and sometimes that works. Maybe you can't rest totally but can put off optional things until later. Maybe you can rest at least one of the first three days of your bleeding. Some women wear special jewelry or clothes to signify they are bleeding to their family & friends, which allows those in their life to give them extra care & extra space. Some women seclude themselves while they bleed.   Some cut back on work those days. Women can honor each other when they are bleeding by helping each other with food, herb teas, massages, taking the kids. I can attest that the investment of time off during bleeding will pay off in more energy to accomplish things during the rest of your cycle.

*   Keep your Exercise very mild - Avoid strenuous exercise = NOT jogging, jumping, running, riding, inverted hatha yoga poses. Excess exercise now can push toxins back into your body, leading to possible diseases later. Gentle stretching or special yoga for menstrual cycle are indicated.

*   Let yourself Turn Inward as much of your bleeding time as possible. The traditional Moon Hut where women secluded themselves during their moon blood was a place where women could be free from daily work & distraction and allow their intuitions & visions to emerge uninterrupted. Use your favorite help to turn inward - meditation, contemplation,   chanting/singing/drumming,   dancing, divination, prayer.

*   Eat a diet to pacify your constitution, eating lightly and warmly (no cold drinks or foods). By eating light, easy to digest food now you allow the energy to go to cleansing rather than digesting new food. Cooked is better than raw. Homemade soups are ideal.

* Handle cravings comfortably - if you crave sweets, eat healthy sweets or just a little organic dark chocolate.

* Shower or bathe with warm water (not very hot or cold). Extremes of temperature can affect the new egg now beginning to mature for release at the next ovulation — especially important if you want to conceive.

* Avoid vigorous massage especially of head. This disturbs the energies wanting to go downward at this time.

• Avoid sexual activity during bleeding time. According to many traditional teachings, intercourse during menses may lead to disease. Low resistance of genital organs during menses means viral infections e.g. herpes may be more easily obtained. Western medicine agrees that there may be a connection between intercourse during menses and endometriosis.

Intercourse during menses can disturb the direction of apana vayu (see section on The Subdoshas) and may create vata abnormality in women's reproductive system.

• Always avoid excessive holding back or forcing of the urge to urinate or defecate to protect apana vayu, the downward moving Vata which rules menses, childbirth, urination & defecation.

* Use external absorbent pads if possible. Tampons create anti peristaltic movements, disturbing the apana vayu. (Also note the possibility of toxic shock syndrome if tampons are left in too long.)

I believe that feeling of the flow coming out of the yoni may be an experience keyed into our inherited physical well-being. Women have been experiencing the sensation of the flow since the beginning of womanhood.

Tampons also encourage the idea that we can just act "normal" during our periods without any possible sign that we are bleeding.

A recent warning was given by one physician that tampons also encourage micro abrasions in the yoni which can leave it more vulnerable to various infections.

Fertility Health

In preparing for a pregnancy, the wise woman & her mate first determine that they are as healthy & in tune as possible. As stated in the chapter "Primer on Ayurveda", the constitution of the coming child is greatly affected by the state of both parents at the time of conception, as well as the environment of the mother's womb during pregnancy. By clearing up any disease or imbalance before pregnancy the best conception and pregnancy possible will be provided. This gives the child a stronger constitution.

After determining their constitutions & their current conditions, the appropriate means are taken to assist the parents-to-be to balance and heal through suitable lifestyle, diet, herbs & pancha karma(purification & rejuvenation practices) whenever possible.

Pancha Karma is useful for deep preparation. Several days of oiling & sweating is used to loosen the toxins in the tissues of the body, followed by appropriate purification & rejuvenation practices under the supervision of a trained Ayurvedic practitioner. Vata imbalance or constitution is balanced with therapeutic & calming bastis (enemas). Pitta imbalance or constitution is balanced by purgation with herbs or yogic methods. Kapha imbalance or constitution is balanced by purgation or (under supervision) therapeutic vomiting. Then rasayana (rejuvenating herbs) are chosen according to need and given to nourish the cleansed tissues. By these means the parents-to-be prepare themselves to receive the soul of their child-to-be in the best possible way.

In addition, parents-to-be can prepare by contemplating, surrounding & filling themselves with the thoughts

& feelings they wish their child to embody. A soul with that energy will then be attracted to them. One story from India illustrates this:

A king was anxious to produce an heir to his throne. However, his wife was a very pious woman who spent all her spare time praying and meditating. When his sons were born they had the temperaments of priests rather than of rulers of the land! Finally she agreed to spend her pregnancy following the day of the king—in court, settling disputes, and meeting with military leaders, training in martial arts. Their next son was well suited to rule the kingdom when it was time for his father to retire.

Requirements for a Healthy Conception

Proper timing gives us the ideal conception time to avoid imbalances being passed on to the child. For Vata parents it's best to conceive in summer & spring, avoiding the fall. For Pitta parents it's best to conceive in spring & winter, avoiding the summer. For Kapha parents it's best to conceive in the fall, avoiding winter & spring. When parents are of mixed doshas then it's best to avoid the mother being out of balance and it is more important to do some preconception balancing.

Another teaching about timing is to never make love on an eclipse, especially when trying to conceive. Meditate, pray, and do work on your subtle levels. An eclipse turns the energy away from the material world, making it unsuitable for starting the manifestation of children or other earthly projects.

Using fertility awareness a woman can be sure of when she is actually ovulating, and is, therefore, fertile. Not all women follow the mid-cycle ovulation average. Sometimes by following the body signals, a woman who was previously frustrated in her tries for pregnancy can achieve her wish through this kind of proper timing. On the other hand, some couples become so obsessed with tracking the cycle that it adds stress to their lives, countering a healthy state for conception. Balance is in order here.

In western astrology it is also possible to add another dimension to choosing a time for conception, according to the angle of the moon at the time the mother was born. For more information on Astrological Fertility Cycles contact Jyoti Wind, astrologer. She has had good results with this added to other techniques for conception. (See the "Resources & Reading List" chapter for her contact information.)

The ground for healthy conception is a healthy uterus and mother. Avoid conception when vaginal infections, herpes or other uterine abnormalities exist in the woman or prostitis, urethritis, or venereal diseases exist in the man. Uterine abnormalities, such as infantile uterus or bifid uterus (needs surgery), retroverted uterus (uterine adjustment needed), fibroids, endometriosis, endometritis, or blocked fallopian tubes are examples. Deal with these problems before conception whenever possible.

Arvigo Techniques of Maya Abdominal Massage® is very useful to help properly position the uterus—it may take some time to move a retroverted uterus, so best not to wait until the month you hope to conceive to seek treatment. This massage also helps to increase circulation in the area & release emotions held there.

Rejuvenative herbs can be used to strengthen the mother if there are no problems present.

The moisture needed for healthy conception is the healthy female egg. The ripening egg begins its development during the previous menses, giving further importance to maintaining balance during the menses. A woman's eggs are all with her even when she is still in her mother's womb prenatally—so they can be affected by any strong imbalances throughout her life. The Arvigo Techniques of Maya Massage® helps here with the circulation of fresh blood and ridding the body of stagnation in the pelvic area.

The seed needed is healthy male seed/sperm. Healthy sperm/semen is slightly sweet smelling, neither extremely thick or stringy or discolored. Imbalance in the semen implies less than optimal sperm. This is best resolved before conception. Spermatogenesis may be increased by the use of various herbs, if this aspect is a problem. Arvigo Techniques of Maya Massage® is useful again for the male to stimulate healthy circulation of blood, lymph and energy for optimal sperm.

Both egg & sperm will be affected by diet & lifestyle at time of ovulation, thus effecting the baby's constitution. During ovulation be especially careful to avoid unsuitable activities, foods or eating habits for your system when inviting a pregnancy to happen.

The Act of Conception

Making love to conceive a child is a sacred act. Meditate & visualize the desired child during making love. Attract the soul you want by setting the stage. A picture of a happy baby is always appropriate. Holy pictures in the room will send a spiritual message to the soul entering the sperm & egg, while a military ambiance would lead to conception of a warrior child.

How to hit the mark? Excessive intercourse can weaken the ojas or vital force of the parents, which can, in turn weaken the ojas and immune system of the child-to-be. Excessive intercourse can also lead to a diminished sperm count. Even medical sources only recommend intercourse every three days when trying to conceive. Through fertility awareness the couple can focus their intercourse timing to when a wished result will occur, rather than expending their vital forces through daily sex for long periods of time. (It's suggested that if there has been no ejaculation for weeks, that the male allows for one ejaculation preconception to remove old sperm before the union leading to conception.)

If drugs of any kind, including alcohol, are used during conception it may lead to less than optimum child. The woman wanting to conceive should avoid over- eating, fasting, or thirst. She should not try to conceive when frightened, dejected, grieving, angry or in love with someone other than the intended father. These states may block conception or the baby conceived may have defects from them.

The ideal time for intercourse according to Ayurveda is between 9 pm - 11 pm. Daytime intercourse tends to weakened kidneys for the sex partners. Midnight intercourse weakens livers of the sex partners. Dawn intercourse can lead to weakened colons.

Various postures are said lead to energy imbalance in the woman. Generally, positioned on her back is considered most balanced in this respect. Breathing through specific nostrils during conception leads to a male or female child.

Through healthy menstrual self care, preconception preparations and conscious conception the best possible start is given to a coming child. Ayurvedic practices have been used for millennia for this very purpose.

Using Susun Weed's Steps of Healing

I was introduced to the Steps of Healing by Susun Weed by her book **Menopausal Years- Wise Woman Ways**. In this book she talks about the menopausal process, using the Steps of Healing as a framework to avoid the all or nothing choices in treatment that the mainstream medical model offers us. The Steps of Healing offer us just that— steps we can take towards health rather than jumping immediately to the most interventive modes of care.

At a workshop I attended with her in Boulder, CO, Susun Weed talked further about the Steps of Healing. She explained that different steps could be seen as different slopes down a mountain. The early steps are very gentle slopes, meandering pathways that may take some time, easy to navigate safely and often very pleasant. The later steps are steeper, maybe shorter—we get down quicker, straighter but increasing side effects of increasing consequences are more frequent.

Because of this, we want to work with the gentle whenever possible. Yet, as she wisely pointed out, there are times of emergency, when speed is of the essence to preserve life. So in some situations we might try the early steps for only a short moment, or do ALL of the Steps of Healing at the same time. After using Steps 5-7 she suggested winding downward again through the steps to cover all the bases, to offer the body all the different qualities of nourishment so that it will recover from the extremes.

For more about Susun and her work go to www.susunweed.com. She also offers a monthly enewsletter, with archives full of useful information.

Steps of Healing for Fertility Enhancement

(Elaborated by Terra from the Steps for Wisewoman Healing by Susun Weed, see more about this renowned herbalist and her Steps of Healing at www.susunweed.com)

0. Do nothing; return to the creative void & do not interfere with the process as it unfolds.

- Meditate

1. Collect information; retrieve from your inner wisdom, ask people, consult oracles, read books.

- Learn Fertility Awareness to be aware of your fertile time - reserve sex for times when you are fertile
- Check for astrological fertility times in your lives
- Read books on conception: Conscious Conception by Jeannine Parvati Baker; Wisewoman Herbal for the Childbearing Year by Susun Weed
- Explore what qualities you desire in your child-to-be & begin living them yourselves
- Discuss what the gifts are of not having a child & being thankful for those; and what the gifts are of having a child.
- Learn about nourishing yourself & maintaining early pregnancy
- Consider the care possibilities available for pregnancy care & birthing

2. Utilize energy or environment; engage elemental forces, walk, bathe, move, breathe.

- Flower essences for enhancing fertility =

- o Alpine lily-positive experience of re-productive organs & ability to con-ceive & sustain pregnancy;
- o Easter lily-cleansing of sexual or-gans, esp. when conception blocked;
- o Forget-me-not - contacting the in-carnating spi-rit;
- o Mariposa lily- bonding w/the in-coming child;
- o Mullein- deciding whether to carry a child;
- o Star tulip- to build trust in one's own mother instincts & encourage inner receptivity;
- o Yellow star tulip - developing tele-pathic com-munication with child;
- o Manzanita - experiencing the body as the spiritual temple of the incar-nating soul
- Lead a lifestyle & eat in a way to avoiding excesses of doshas
- Use chanting of holy names to invoke spiri-tual energy
- Wear white clothes, white garlands
- Drink vital waters; walk on the earth, lean on trees, bathe in sunlight, moonlight, practice breath work all to invoke the natural elemen-tal forces

3. Nourish & tone; nourish yourself optimally, open to compassion

- Eat ojas increasing diet = dairy, ghee, sattvic foods, shatavari, ashwagunda, guduchi; Ojas increasing practices include meditation; chanting Om & sexual moderation; avoid ojas decreasing factors such as anger, hunger, worry, sorrow & overwork; excesssive sexual activity, stress, anxiety, devitalized food, unnatural environment & lifestyle

- Nourishing herbs & rasayanas = chyvan prash/ shakti prana; shatavari, ashwagunda, red raspberry, oatstraw, nettles, red clover, alfalafa
- Eat concentrated nutritional foods according to your doshas to add nutrition to your body = blue-green algae, sea vegetables, bee pollen, wheat germ, sunflower seeds, pumpkin seeds
- Massage & energy work – Arvigo Techniques of Maya Abdominal Massage® , Reiki, Jin Shin, Polarity

4. Stimulate & sedate; use herbs to facilitate desired effect (remember to work w/doshas & know the herbs or consult w/practitioner before using!)

- Herbs that increase spermatogenesis = brahmi; shatavari; vidari; jatamansi; garlic; onion; sucanat; ginseng; ghee; milk; banana; 1/2 tsp amalaka + 1 tsp ghee + 1/2 tsp honey; 1 tsp ashwagunda w/ 1 cup milk morning & night; gokshur; pippili w/fennel; rose; white sugar water; prabhav nasya & 1 tsp orally;
- Herbs that increase female fertility = 1/2 tsp amalaki + 1 tsp ghee + 1/2 tsp honey; mace; manjistha; saffron; shatavari; vidari
- Herbs that increase sexual desire = tulsi increases love; 2 hrs after lunch/dinner or 1 hr before dinner or breakfast eat 1 banana + 1 tsp warm ghee + 1 tsp sucanat + pinch cardamon powder will keep sexual energy high for hours according to Dr.Vasant Lad; hot

garlic milk; 1 tsp ashwagunda w/ 1 cup milk 90 min before making love

5. Use drugs; vitamin & mineral supplements, immediate results.

- Fertility enhancing drugs - ex. clomid increases female ovulation
- Male enhancement drugs such as Viagra®
- Artificially controlling the fertility cycle of the woman by using exogenous hormones
- Artificial insemination

6. Break & enter; use invasive technology that forcefully enters the physical, emotional or energetic body

- Surgical removal of eggs, external fertilization of egg & surgical implantation of embryo
- Frozen embryos, frozen sperm

Snapshots of Vata-Pitta-Kapha in Fertility

Snapshots are just that—a picture of one moment, from one angle of a dynamic situation. There might be more doshas involved. Tissue damage may have occurred. These lists are to give you a feel for out of balance doshas in the various phases of the childbearing year. They do not imply that just drinking some tea will correct them. Always seek appropriate care.

Excess Vata in Fertility
- Irregular menstrual cycles
- Lack of fertile mucus
- Lack of development of the uterine lining
- Lack of ovulation
- Uterine scarring or adhesions post surgery
- Blockage of fallopian tubes due to previous PID
- Blockage of cervix by scarring from cervical tearing, cervical freezing, laser, cone biopsy
- Miscarriage
- Too thin
- Dyspareunia
- >40 years old
- Malpositioned of the uterus

Soothing Vata for Fertility
- Individualized evaluation and program to balance Vata and stimulate circulation with Arvigo Techniques of Maya Abdominal Massage® (ATMAM).
- Castor oil and massage for physical blockage. May require surgical intervention if natural doesn't work.

Excess Pitta in Fertility
- Vaginal infections
- Allergy to partner's semen & sperm
- Excessive bleeding with menses
- Excessive acidity of vaginal fluids- hostile to sperm
- Endometriosis
- Irritability of uterine lining
- Pelvic Inflammatory Disease(PID)
- Overproduction of androgens

Soothing Pitta for Fertility
- Treatment of infections
- Individualized evaluation and program to balance Pitta along with ATMAM® to stimulate circulation once the infection is treated

Excess Kapha in Fertility
- Yeast infections
- Stagnation
- Underactive thyroid
- Overweight or obese
- Submucosal fibroids
- Endometrial polyps
- Diabetes

Soothing Kapha for Fertility
- Individualized evaluation and program to balance Kapha including ATMAM® to stimulate circulation.

Supporting Pregnancy with Ayurveda

Pregnancy is a very special season in the life of a woman. Tremendous changes happen within -- physically, mentally, emotionally, and spiritually. There is a tendency in our culture for women to ignore their pregnancy (just as they try to ignore their menstrual/fertility cycles) and act as though there is nothing different about them except that there's a baby growing inside.

Ayurvedic teachings promote a proper attitude of worship towards all pregnant women. They are fulfilling the very important full time role of bringing new life into the world. Their experiences in pregnancy directly feed into the sensory & mental organs of the developing child—so the more beautiful, loving, and uplifting the mother's experience, the healthier the child will tend to perceive and think about the world throughout his or her life. Wise women give themselves all the space & time possible to turn inward during their pregnancies, to listen to their bodies & their intuitions, and to tune in to the beneficent forces available to them in the physical & spiritual worlds. In this way they give birth with grace and their children are blessed with the best possible start in the world.

Energetically, pregnancy is full of change, creativity,& expansion, so Vata is normally emphasized. Metabolism & warmth in the body is increased so Pitta is normally increased. And the bulk of the body is increased so Kapha is also normally increased. In each woman these changes are interplaying with her constitution, the baby's constitution, and her environmental influences. The intricacy of working with pregnant women is further increased by the need to avoid any therapies and herbs which may disturb the uterus and the apana prana or downward energy.

The apana prana is key to maintaining the pregnancy as well as naturally birthing the baby at the time of labor. This emphasizes the utility of taking care of imbalanced conditions before pregnancy whenever possible, since it is generally more complex to treat women during pregnancy. Prevention is emphasized for self care, with treatment generally reserved to experienced Ayurvedic practitioners.

General Recommendations for Pregnancy Self-Care

Eat and follow lifestyle according to current Ayurvedic condition rather than strictly by constitution. This is because the baby's needs & desires start being felt more by the mother in her food preferences and energetics especially after the 5th month - satisfy cravings while maintaining discrimination; eat fresh food, avoiding processed or leftover food, refined sugars, very spicy foods, food straight from the refrigerator or freezer, and chemical additives in foods

Nutritional needs are increased during pregnancy - quantity as well as quality. The need for more calories, calcium, protein, & iron is noteworthy. Nourishing herbal infusions can help fulfill these needs - for Pitta & Kapha: Red Raspberry &/or Nettles; for Vata : Oatstraw . The pregnant woman can drink up to a quart daily suitable for her type, 1-2 cups of other infusions. To make an infusion : put a big handful of herbs in quart jar, fill with boiling hot water, & let it sit 4-6 hours. Strain & refrigerate what you don't drink immediately. You can rewarm it as needed. Organic herbs are always the best choice. (Avoid herbs unsafe for pregnancy!-See)
Nutritional Ayurvedic herbs & preparations are also good: ghee; chyvan prash VK- P+ for cold season; and

shakti prana VPK- for hot season or if high P (see "Resources & Reading List" chapter for where to get herbs).

Eating is only the first step. **Digesting** is equally important. Signs of poor digestion are gas, belching, stomach & intestinal discomforts. Rules for good digestion are the same in pregnancy as at other times. See the chapter "Caring for Digestion" for specific rules. In addition:
- Cooked, moist soupy & warm foods are generally easier to digest than raw.
- Adding digestive herbs to food may help digestion.

Ayurvedic digestive herbs safe for pregnancy include - mints; pippili, tarragon; cardamom; jasmine; cumin; cinnamon; basil.

Other digestive helps – papaya (be aware that digestive enzymes may be Pitta provoking on a long term basis). A substitute would be Agni Kindler (see "Recipe" chapter for how to make this) Agni Kindler will stimulate one's own digestive enzymes into action, rather than adding others artificially. To help with absorption of nutrients, drink takram after meals. This recipe is also found in "Recipe" chapter.

Happiness & love are true nourishment for mother & the baby. Ways to increase these elements of your life are:
- Worship, chant, pray, meditate
- Contemplate the lives of saints & other great beings
- Be with people who uplift you
- Avoid disturbing TV or violent movies and books
- Have as beautiful & peaceful an environment as possible
- Eat only fresh whole foods.

The mate is an important part of the process. The mate's time, energy, & nourishing of the mother are important to the development of the baby. Ayurveda recognizes that marital problems during pregnancy can even physically affect the baby - so nurturing the marital relationship nurtures the baby & strengthens the safe haven it will be born into.

Ayurvedic fetal development teachings tell us that the constitution of the baby is formed by the genetic makeup of mother & father; the diet & emotions of the mother during pregnancy; environmental influences; and the samskaras or spiritual patterns that the soul brings in with it from previous incarnations. Ayurveda teaches that the baby is physically conscious of his or her development, which is being confirmed today by the science of perinatal psychology.

One important teaching is that what the mother takes in through HER sense organs goes into the development of the baby's sense organs. This further emphasizes the importance of what kind of environment the woman is in during pregnancy. There were even traditional ceremonies for different stages of pregnancy to "feed" the specific senses. Today we can emphasize as much as possible that the pregnant woman see beautiful & loving things, listen to loving & melodious sounds, touch pleasing things & be touched in loving ways, taste wholesome tastes, and smell fragrant odors during pregnancy.

During the first 2 months only astral projection connects the baby to its current body. The 4th month is VERY CRITICAL- the heart starts to develop as the seat of consciousness. This leads to the baby's desires starting to express themselves through the mother's desires. If mother has a hard time with husband during this month, the baby's heart may develop defects. After this time the mental body becomes connected to the physical body.

In the eighth month **ojas (vital fluid)** moves from mother to the baby. Creating and conserving ojas is especially important at this time. Ways to build ojas include:

- Being sure your digestion is working well.
- Eating more ojas producing foods: ghee, milk, dates, apricots, sesame seeds, almonds, Ayurvedic tonics such as ashwagunda or shatavari which are in many nutritive Ayurvedic jams.
- Being more inward-- stay at home & rest more than usual at this time to ensure good vitality for both mother & baby.
- Spend time in nature.
- Chant OM.
- Be in touch with Divinity in your own way.
- Meditate.

What to avoid to conserve ojas: anger, worry, overwork, drugs or stimulants, hunger, sorrow, excessive sex, and devitalized food.

Rubbing **warm sesame oil on the soles of the feet** to helps balance Vata and also stimulates the energy points of the feet, keeping energy flowing throughout the body. A great way to unwind & to spend quiet time together is for mates to regularly give evening foot massages to each other. (sesame oil may be too "hot" for Pittas - almond oil might be better for them)

Avoid sleeping in the day to avoid causing imbalances, especially for Kapha people—unless you are not sleeping well at night and become Vata. Resting is beneficial at the right times & in the right amounts for personal needs.

Daily walks or swims are **appropriate exercise**, as well as yoga asanas indicated for pregnancy. Gentle stretching of the pelvis helps flexibility during labor. I recommend the book Active Birth by Janet Balaskas for exercises. Avoid overly vigorous exercise, & exercise where injury is more likely, such as skiing or horseback riding. Jarring exercises can disturb the apana vayu. Never exercise to full capacity! This depletes ojas/ immune & vital force, so key to building the baby's future health as well as that of the mother.

Taking **warm baths** relaxes muscles when feeling tense. Tension inhibits circulation, thus movement of both blood and energy. It keeps toxins locked in the body rather than moving them out. Full body massage of a proper nature is very healthy, allowing the woman to integrate her body changes, while relaxing her and benefiting her physiology.

Aromatherapy can be helpful also as part of tension relief-- be sure to use only oils indicated safe for pregnancy!!!
Essential Oils Generally Considered Safe in Pregnancy

Tangerine; Mandarin; Grapefruit; Geranium; Roman Chamomile, Rose Bulgar; Rose Maroc; Jasmine; Ylang-ylang; Lavender

Pelvic floor exercises (Kegels) tone & strengthen the muscles of the pelvic floor - which during pregnancy must support the weight of the baby, as well as the uterus & bladder. They also help regulate the apana. These exercises are good for pelvic health throughout the life cycle, increasing strength, circulation & health of tissues for greater orgasms as well as continued health through the elder years.

Once you know Kegels practice, anywhere, anytime - even the grocery line!!! Tighten the sling of muscles holding up the internal pelvic organs, from the pubic bone back to the tailbone. You can practice tightening the whole muscle first. Be sure that you are not just contracting your abdominal or buttocks muscles—focus on moving only the inward muscles It may help to practice lying down first to relieve some pressure and build up to standing/sitting ones. Do each 200x/day, slowly or quickly, in rounds of 10 building up to rounds of 20. Or try elevator kegels, which tighten upward in 3 levels and then go back down 3 levels. Talk with your midwife or a physical therapist about doing this properly. As you become more aware of this muscle you can work on the more specific areas.

Bladder-Strengthening exercise- Practice tightening & releasing the muscles that control urine flow from the bladder. Do this once when peeing to find the muscles, then practice it away from urination. Continual interruption of urination may lead to bladder infections.

Vaginal exercise- Try tightening & releasing the muscles of the vagina around a finger or a penis to find the vaginal muscles. Then do rounds of 10 building up to 20 at a time.

Anal Sphincter exercise- known in yoga as Ashwini mudra: This energy exercise helps balance Vata & the apana prana energy, especially useful in pregnancy. Directions - in a quiet place, eyes closed —Inhale completely & (if not pregnant) hold the breath. Contract & release the anal sphincter rapidly & repeatedly. Hold the breath only so long as the following exhalation can be slow & controlled. Begin with three rounds of about 10 pulls each. Don't bear down when holding the breath, which could strain ligaments & put downward pressure on the uterus. Repeat daily.

Avoid overly vigorous sex, especially at the usual times when menses would be expected or if there are any signs that the pregnancy is fragile (spotting or cramping or lots of low pressure). Sexual excesses may also use up ojas or cause doshic imbalances, especially of apana prana which can cause many different problems of pregnancy & birth. Women are more susceptible to infections at this time too. Ayurveda traditionally encourages celibacy during pregnancy. Doing yoga asanas, pranayama & meditation are traditional ways to naturally control sexual desires through spiritual practice. The most important factors if continuing an active sexual life is to do so in a loving context & with awareness of what feels comfortable & right to the woman.

Beginning the 8th month, begin to apply licorice ghee to vagina. (available from the Ayurvedic herbalist, Louise Sanchez, listed in "Resources & Reading List" chapter.) **Perineal massage** 4-5x week will make the tissues healthy & supple, allowing them to stretch readily for the birthing of the baby. It also helps women get used to the unusual sensation of their vagina stretching to birth a baby so that they can relax at that point & be less likely to tear or to slow down the pushing stage to keep from being over-whelmed with sensations or emotions. It usually works best for the mate to do it for the woman, but if that's not possible she can try stretch herself (on the toilet or lying on your side may work easier in this case).

Directions: Wash hands, then use the licorice ghee as lubricant insert one or two fingers along the bottom of the vagina. After a couple of inches there is a "drop-off" where the inner edge of the muscles lie. Massage the whole bottom half of this vaginal sling gently yet firmly enough to create a definite stretching, burning sensation. Along with the massage, the woman should practice relaxing these muscles, while they are being stretched to their limit. Over a week or two there often is a noticeable change in stretchabil-ity. Continue gently pushing the limit of stretching & relaxing until the birth.

Traditionally, in the last month of pregnancy the woman may be given small, gentle therapeutic oil enemas to be sure that the **apana prana is balanced for the work of labor**. Consult with an Ayurvedic Practitioner before doing this for directions and to be sure it is appropriate After this process the woman nearing labor eats a predominantly Vata reducing diet, adjusted to her needs & the season. The emphasis is on preventing an imbalance of the apana prana which can lead to malposition or uterine malfunction during labor. At the very least, avoid holding back urine, gas, or bowel movements; getting chilled; or getting jarred to support the proper movement of the apana.

The **proper caregiver** is important during pregnancy, birth & postpartum. This person should be both technically knowledgeable & open-hearted. The woman must feel comfortable with this person -- they will share the intimate moments of giving birth and be one of the first people the baby will relate to. If the birthing woman doesn't feel relaxed, up-lifted & trusting of this person it can impede the labor process, possibly leading to complications. Wise women pick someone familiar with many forms of healing which can be used before resorting to drugs & surgery as solutions. Complete pregnancy care includes nutritional counseling and time to get questions answered & concerns addressed.

Steps of Healing Self-Inquiries for Pregnancy

These are suggestions for ways to take care of yourself between pregnancy visits and it also is information useful to your midwives in helping you take care of yourself - these are things they would like to know about you.

(Elaborated by Terra from the Steps for Wisewoman Healing by Susun Weed, see more at www.susunweed.com)

0. Do nothing; return to the creative void & do not interfere with the process as it unfolds.

1. Collect information; retrieve from your inner wisdom, ask people, consult oracles, read books.
- Describe your general state of well-being.
- Since the last pregnancy visit have you experienced any problems? illnesses? complaints? Please list them & if you have done something about it, what you did.
- Have you seen any kind of health practition-ers?
- Describe the baby & its movements since the last visit.
- How are your family relationships, work situations, living situation since last visit?
- Any special dreams or omens?
- Any fears, joys, questions you need answered?
- Any special stresses?
- Have you read any books about birth, etc.?

2. Utilize energy or environment; engage elemental forces, walk, bathe, move, breathe.
- How much time out-of-doors?
- What kind & how much exercise? Kegels?

- How have you paid attention to the baby?
- How are you experiencing your sexual energy?
- Taking relaxing baths & invigorating showers?
- Have you kept the energy flowing well w/ midwives by keeping payment & other agreements?

3. Nourish & tone; nourish mother & baby optimally, open to compassion
- Are you getting enough hugs & snuggles?
- Are you drinking nourishing herbal infusions daily?
- How much alone time have you been having?
- How much sleep have you had lately & what quality?
- Any massage or energy work? Perineal & butt massage?
- Describe three days of your eating habits on the back of this sheet - pick one average day, one above average day & one below average day.

4. Stimulate & sedate; use herbs to facilitate desired effect, initiate and move forward, slow down and reset the clock.
- Have you used any herbs to stimulate or sedate yourself?
- 5. Use drugs; vitamin & mineral supplements, immediate results.
- Have you taken any over-the-counter or prescription drugs? Medicinal herbs? Food supplements? If so, please list them.

6. Break & enter; use invasive technology that forcefully enters the physical, emotional or energetic body

Snapshots of Vata-Pitta-Kapha in Pregnancy

Excess Vata in Pregnancy
- Late to appointments
- Changeable appetite, irregular eating habits
- Thin, may be very tall or very short, lack of fat tissue
- Dry skin, dry mucus membranes-dehydration possible
- Nervous, overwhelmed, traumatized in past/easily now as well
- Tendency to fear reactions
- Talks incessantly, wiggles her foot, taps fingers, twists hair—can't sit still
- Absent minded- forgets to eat, drink; learns easily but forgets quickly too
- Has trouble following through on recommendations due to distraction
- Worries over everything
- May over exercise, go to extremes, lack of routine
- Erratic growth during pregnancy
- Tendency to malpositioning of baby due to her lack of muscle tone
- Elderly primagravida (age tends to increase Vata in everyone)
- Tends to wake around 3 am, with difficulty going back to sleep
- Creative artist-artisan

Soothing Vata in Pregnancy

- Be calm and grounded yourself to transmit this to this sensitive woman.
- Gentle touch can be soothing- slow, repetitive, encompassing, steady
- Self massage with warm sesame or almond oil can be very soothing- especially the feet and the head
- Use gentle speech and focus on positive languaging, avoiding comments that might scare her
- Write down her homework from your visits with her.
- Encourage routine in her life, especially for eating, sleeping, BM
- Have a routine in your visits with her, so she knows what to expect, and so, can inwardly relax
- Diet must include plenty of high quality protein (to ground her) avoiding beans
- Include healthy oils such as virgin olive oil, ghee, butter, coconut oil. Fish oil or flax/hemp oil for EFAs is important.
- Avoid raw foods- more cooked, moist, oiled foods
- Avoid left overs, foods warmed in microwave
- An ideal Vata soothing meal- soup with root vegetables, some kind of meat, broth, ghee or olive oil, mild spices and salt to taste.
- Good nourishing herb for strengthening her body and nervous system – oat straw infusions

Excess Pitta in Pregnancy

- Allergies
- Irritable, angry, critical
- Anemia beyond normal
- Liver problems/Toxicity – morning sickness, preeclampsia
- Overworking and ambitious
- Competitive
- Control issues
- Red hair
- Average sized, average growth
- Bleeding tendencies
- Heartburn with strong digestion
- Demands respect
- Follows recommendations well, if she convinced it is in her best interest
- May have trouble going to sleep

Soothing Pitta in Pregnancy

- Raw sweet fruit and green vegetables good, with whole grains
- Good herbal infusion for balancing Pitta is nettles.
- An ideal Pitta meal- green salad with lime juice dressing, lentil pilaf, and blueberries for dessert.
- Moon light, being by bodies of water or even a fountain
- Cool it!   Less ambition, less work, fewer projects
- Avoid hot spicy foods, tomatoes,
- Explain everything with lots of evidence, logic and reason

Excess Kapha in Pregnancy

- Weight gain excessive
- Fluid retention
- Excess mucus or congestion
- Yeast infections
- Rarely exercises
- In denial
- Slow to change
- May sleep excessively

Soothing Kapha in Pregnancy
- Avoid dairy products, especially cold ones and sweets
- Eat light, nourishing, spicier foods, mostly vegetables and protein
- An ideal meal for Kapha is whole wheat pita bread with humus and vegetables in it.
- Nourishing herbal infusion for Kapha is nettles or red raspberry.
- Exercise every day
- Stimulation of the mind and body is good to avoid stagnation

Ayurvedic Helps for Some Pregnancy Discomforts

Morning sickness –
Determine the origin of the nausea symptoms by looking at the other symptoms the woman has in her body and mind and her pulse= Vata (Prana/Udana), Pitta, or Kapha. Seek advanced help if severe, dehydration, or past the first trimester.

Prana/Udana type- This is appropriate if less than 10 incidents of vomiting have occurred. Dry roast BLACK cardamom seeds and then powder them. Use 1 tsp of the powder in the morning,(with milk, if that's possible). DO NOT USE GREEN CARDAMOM-it can cause miscarriage.

Pitta type-
Use shatavari, the female tonic and Pitta reducing herb: roast in an iron pan ghee w/ cardamom & date sugar

To increase digestion –
See Caring for Digestion chapter

Anemia –
True anemia is a Pitta problem, physiologic anemia due to blood volume expansion near the end of pregnancy isn't.
- Punanarva mandura tablets
- Brahmi ghee
- Food sources of iron

Constipation –
- 1 cup hot spiced cows milk w/ 1 tsp ghee before bed (use spices according to your doshas)

- Use a little amalaki is OK, esp. if high Pitta or Vata & Pitta provoked.

Hyperacidity w/ coated tongue –
This is Pitta condition. Use general Pitta soothing.
- Figs
- Small pinch amalaki

Heartburn , allergies –
These are Pitta conditions. Use Pitta soothing regime, especially avoiding high Pitta foods.
- Coriander,
- Shatavari,
- Pinch of amalaki

Insomnia --
Treat according to dosha with diet, lifestyle &-
- Vata-(wake 3 am or after with trouble going back to sleep) – massage soles of feet with warm sesame oil & ashwaganda – ½ tsp in warmcow or rice milk at bedtime
- Pitta –(trouble going to sleep or waking around midnight)—shatavari powder – 1 tsp in warm milk or rice milk at bedtime

Ayurvedic tonics –
These are tasty mixes of nutritive and rejuvenative herbs with ghee and honey. Take 1 tsp daily on empty stomach, 15 min later 1 cup warm milk or water
- chyvan prash (cold season or after a respiratory sickness)
- shakti prana (hot season or P+),

Check Chapter on Resources and Reading List for where to order herbs. For more on the discomforts of pregnancy –
The Wisewoman Herbal for the Childbearing Year by Susun Weed for western herbal helps, along with
The Yoga of Herbs by Lad & Frawley to check them according to dosha.

Supporting Labor and Birth with Ayurveda

Traditionally, most births were taken care of by the midwives rather than Ayurvedic physicians. Because of this, many of the teachings about labor & birth are not written down in the texts (which were written by men) but passed on orally from midwife to apprentice. The physicians only dealt with the most complicated situations.

Ancient texts do talk about having special spaces for giving birth which would take into account the spiritual as well as practical needs. When the woman is showing signs of beginning labor she would enter the birth space with special blessings & ceremony, to mark the significance of this time. She would be accompanied by birth attendants that were calm & supportive, inspiring the confidence of the birthing woman.

To awaken and balance the apana prana for early labor, an enema of dashamula tea can be used. To help keep balance of the Vata energy which is very high at this time, the woman must avoid becoming chilled. Massaging her with warm oil & giving her a warm bath, as well as feeding her broths & soups, avoiding icy cold drinks or foods can be useful for maintaining balance of Vata & apana prana.

Marma points (Ayurvedic energy points) can be massaged firmly with circular motion for about 5 minutes with clary sage essential oil to encourage labor and mix the clary sage with rose to soothe pain.

To encourage labor –
Bhaga - the midpoint of the pubic bone
Nabhi - points halfway between navel and each crest of pelvic bones
Urvi - midpoint on posterior and anterior aspects of thigh

For pain in labor –
Triku – tip of the coccyx (use 2 thumbs)
Manibandha – midpoint of inner wrist
Bhaga – the midpoint of the pubic bone – press for pain

The use of walking and massaging the pelvic area with warm sesame or castor oil will also help the baby move down in labor. All of these Vata/ apana soothing measures are also used to help when there is some malposition of the baby so that it can move more easily through the birth canal.

When the birth of the baby is approaching, licorice ghee is used for perineal massage. After the climax of giving birth, the woman is kept comfortable & warm and fed Vata reducing foods such a stews and soups. The placenta is allowed to deliver most naturally and the cord of to the baby is not cut until ALL pulsation has stopped. This allows the transfer of ojas to the baby to be complete, giving it good vital force & immunity. It can take 1 –2 hours for pulsation of the cord to stop if you feel right next to the baby's tummy on the cord. Measure 8 fingers away from the baby's belly to find where to cut. Traditionally a special knife was used to cut the cord during a ceremony, again marking the ritual significance of the baby being severed from the mother. Antiseptic herbs or oils were used to keep the cord area from infection until healed.

The baby is kept cozy. Warm sesame oil is massaged onto the fontanelles to protect from over stimulation. . A little hat, especially if made of silk, can help as well .

Traditionally babies were gagged to spit up to clear their stomach of anything swallowed during labor..

They were also given special experiences to tune them into their Vedic culture. One was feeding baby honey, ghee & specially prepared edible gold to give the baby a type of Ayurvedic immunization to the local pollens & dairy as well as increased vitality & immunity with the gold. Other properties are also given by the substances – honey clears Kapha which is predominant in children; ghee increases the healthy fat in the brain to increase intellect, as well as nourishing nerve & marrow tissues; and gold signifies wealth. A gold spoon can be used instead of gold preparation, if unavailable.

The baby is massaged with pure oil and bathed in mild herbal bath such as calendula herb. Baby receives breast milk as the best food. Herbs can be used to enhance breast milk formation in the mother — Shatavari, Vidari, Ajwain. Before milk comes in babies are often traditionally fed ghee & honey*, in the amount of a baby handful, just 2-3 times a day.

In this way the baby & mother have gone through the transitional time of pregnancy & childbirth with the nurturance & help of Ayurveda.

* Western medicine says there is a spore in the honey that can cause problems for newborn.

Steps of Healing for Labor & Birth Self Care

Elaborated by Terra from the Steps of Healing by Susun Weed

0. Do nothing; return to the creative void & do not interfere with the process as it unfolds.
- Protect the inherent, continuous bond between mother & baby which guides their birthing process.
- Allow the protective, supportive bond between mother & mate which is the womb of the birthing process to fully function & come to fruition.

1. Collect information; retrieve from your inner wisdom, ask people, consult oracles, read books.
- Tune in to your body, your process, your intuition.
- Tune in to your spiritual guides, your Higher Power..
- Tune in to the baby & its movements, its process, its intuition..
- How are your family relationships, work situations, living situation impacting your laboring/birthing/mothering ?
- Any special dreams or omens?
- Acknowledge fears, joys, angers, questions you need answered, any special stresses
- Consult books /videos about birth, etc..
- Go outside to notice the weather condition. How does it relate?

2. Utilize energy or environment; engage elemental forces, walk, bathe, move, breathe.
- How have you paid attention to the baby?
- Use air - Try some time out-of-doors. let fresh air in the room; use deep, long, relaxed breathing or just

change how you are breathing to go with your intuition; make noises.

- Use fire - light a candle; enhance or dim lights; walk; go up & down stairs; dance; make love.
- Use water - bathe; shower; drink lots of water; use hot compresses &/or cool washcloth to balance your temperature.
- Use earth - stand on the ground; consciously send your energy & your baby down towards Mother Earth.
- Use ether/the intangible - love your baby; love your spouse; use homeopathics, flower remedies, aromatherapy.

3. Nourish & tone; nourish mother & baby optimally, open to compassion
- Are you drinking plenty of nourishing herbal infusions?
- Take alone time.
- Rest & sleep when the time is ripe.
- Use massage &/or energy work.
- Eat what feel right in labor.
- Is it time for hugging or cuddling?

4. Stimulate & sedate; use herbs to facilitate desired effect, initiate and move forward, slow down and reset the clock.
- Have you used anything to stimulate or sedate yourself?

5. Use drugs; vitamin & mineral supplements, immediate results.
- Have you taken any over-the-counter or prescription drugs? Medicinal herbs? Food supplements? If so, please list them. Ex. castor oil; blue/black cohosh; etc.

6. Break & enter; use invasive technology that forcefully enters the physical, emotional or energetic body
- Are you being motivated by fear?
- Do not allow any uninvited or unwelcome interactions.

Snapshots of Vata-Pitta-Kapha in Labor & Birth

Excess Vata during Labor

- Unripe cervix
- Premature rupture of membranes
- Irregular contractions
- Malposition
- Start and stop labor
- Hypotonic contractions
- Dehydration – and associated maternal fever, tachycardia
- Fearfulness, overwhelmed feelings
- Irritable or exhausted uterus leading to lack of progress
- Shoulder dystocia due to malpositioning

Soothing Vata during Labor

- Keep warm, avoiding drafts & chills
- Warm sitz bath or tub bath, being sure not to get chilled when done with them.
- Massage with warm sesame oil (or if signs of ama (toxicity) always use warm castor oil)
- If there's an appetite, eat cooked warm foods and drinks, avoiding cold drinks & foods
- Reduce unnecessary stimulation –reduce cortical stimulation (lowered light, no watchful eyes or too much talking), limit vaginal exams
- Assure hydration with Recharge, miso soup
- Encourage rest

Excess Pitta during Labor – remember that sometimes Vata will push Pitta—such as a fever after rupture of membranes with excess vaginal exams

- Fever

- Precipitous labor
- Hypertonic contractions
- Excess bleeding; postpartum hemorrhage
- Hypoglycemia

Soothing Pitta during Labor
- Assure hydration to flush any extra acidity from uterus and balance any blood loss
- Be sure nourished
- Avoid overheating

Excess Kapha during Labor
- Slow progress due to large baby
- Shoulder dystocia due to excess weight gain
- Cepalopelvic disproportion

Soothing Kapha during Labor – remember that the Kapha woman usually has plenty of stamina, we don't know if the baby is Kapha.
- Keeping active and moving helps overcome stagnation due to Kapha
- The birth attendant must be patient, while stimulating and watchful.

Postpartum Care with Ayurveda

The postpartum is a very tender period of time for mother and baby. Ayurveda's recommendations can protect them from taking on imbalance & stress during this sensitive time. During pregnancy the woman is to be worshipped as a creatrix; postpartum this level of devotion and caring is twice as necessary, for it includes both Mother & Child.

Ayurvedic teachings tell us that postpartum is one of the special times in a woman's life that her whole physiology is changing quickly and can be set to actually rejuvenate the mother. The women I know who have followed these teachings postpartum have had better postpartum experiences and continued to feel better as their life went on. In contrast, most women in our culture try to get back to "normal" life as quickly as possible—it's almost as if it is a sign of strength to act as though postpartum isn't a special time. This is dangerous for the future health of the mother—if she overdoes it and is careless in the weeks following the birth she can be setting up imbalances that can plague her for the rest of her life.

One example of what can happen was "June", an athletic & healthy Pitta woman, who felt great right after her birth – and proceeded to go on long, strenuous hikes just 2 weeks after giving birth. In the year following the birth June found herself getting weaker instead of stronger and having frequent bouts of illness – something which hadn't happened for her before. Only though strong attention to her imbalances that stemmed from postpartum could she rebuild her immune system and strength to withstand the stresses of motherhood.

With postpartum care & attention the picture can look much healthier. "Stacey", a Vata woman, had already given birth once before. During the first postpartum she developed a sleeping problem (Vata type- waking at about 3 am) that stuck with her for years. When she began using Ayurveda she finally cleared up the problem. Then she became pregnant again and was worried she may fall back into the old pattern. However, this time she followed the Ayurvedic postpartum recommendations and she ended up feeling great after her postpartum, with no sleep disorders.

The postpartum period is one generally of great change. The changeable sleep schedule, the loss of fluids common to postpartum, changing hormonal balance, the loss of weight, and the extra space left in the abdomen after childbirth means Vata is there for the mother. Women who went through a cesarean section are even more Vata due to the opening up of their abdomen & uterus, letting air & space into their inner most body. The mothering of a newborn with its irregular and changeable schedule also contributes greatly to Vata dosha easily going out of balance. Vata reducing measures are necessary to prevent Vata symptoms or the possibility of Vata moving any excess Pitta or Kapha in the body to form symptoms of those doshas.

For the baby, leaving the contained and watery womb to go into the spacious, airy, stimulating, and relatively dry world also means a big increase in Vata dosha. The baby is just unfolding into this world, learning to adapt and to act in a dance with life. Introduction of harsh stimuli & separation from the mother during this time are insults to the tender nervous system of the newborn. So during this time Vata reduction is the basic care plan to help both mother & baby.

As mentioned in the first chapter of this book, Vata is made up of space and air. It has the qualities of: dry, cold, light, changeable, mobile, and rough. It's "home base" in the body is the abdominal/pelvic area – so key in childbearing. When it is balanced we express it through living in a flowing, flexible, enthusiastic, and creative way. Some of the symptoms of imbalance are constipation, shakiness, gas, cramps, sleep disturbance and fatigue. Emotional symptoms of Vata imbalance are feelings of being overwhelmed, fearful, and/or distracted. It is also related to grief.

Vata reducing measures counter the qualities of Vata. We use moisture and oiliness, warmth, heaviness, routine, stillness & quiet, and smooth, flowing lifestyle.

Many of these Ayurvedic postpartum teachings were first promoted in our country through the Mother Baby Program of Maharishi Mahesh Yogi and further developed by Ysha (Martha) Oakes, Diplomate Ayurvedic Postpartum Practitioner, Experienced Ayurvedic Postpartum Doula Trainer. If you would like to learn more about training or consult with her, you can reach her at www.sacredwindow.com. She also has a self-published book available expanding on the information in this article, recommended if you want to try it or help others with it.

First of all we must **"Mother the Mother"**. While the new mom is mothering the baby, she too must receive care. In this way both baby & mother are best nurtured. She should not be entertaining visitors, cleaning house, doing laundry, or cooking meals. To the best of their ability, families must plan together ahead of time and in a thorough manner, how to have the mom taken care of for 4-6 weeks postpartum. Most people may not be able to provide care for a full six weeks - at least 2 is a minimum to prevent the mom from doing too much. In our midwifery practice we usually said two weeks minimum with an extra week for each other child in the household.

One danger is that the partner will try to take up all the slack, becoming exhausted too. This can be emotionally as well as physically trying. It is important to call on the community to support the family at this time. Churches, coworkers, friendship circles and support groups are often good places to find this help. If a woman doesn't have this kind of community when she becomes pregnant it is most important to start developing it—it will serve her throughout parenthood.

The pregnant women can ask a friend to coordinate volunteers. They would use a sign-up sheet at the baby shower or blessing way and then the friend would call people after the birth to confirm when they would come by to clean, drop off food, or do some laundry. Specific personal food needs & guidelines are best in writing & given to everyone providing food. Enough food could be supplied for both supper and lunch.

Another time honored technique for mothering the mother is to have family or friends come & stay for some time postpartum. It's imperative that everyone feels absolutely comfortable about the person staying there—or the stress will offset the help provided! Plenty of communication about boundaries needs to be made before, during & after the visit to keep things clear and easy.

Oiliness is needed to offset the dryness and roughness of Vata. This is provided postpartum through daily oil massage with warm sesame oil, eating food with plenty of ghee and olive oil, and sesame oil enemas (only when working with a trained practitioner).

The daily oil massage is best done by someone trained in Ayurvedic postpartum massage—but these practitioners are still few & far between. The technique specially suited to the Vata needs of the women & their changing bodies is a slow, gentle, firm (but not deep), steady, integrative, repetitive massage with warm sesame oil. Plenty of oil to the head is important for calming the nervous system. It's good to have someone there to help with the baby during the massage time and try to schedule so feeding happens just beforehand so mom can relax as deeply as possible – and whoever massages should be ready for the needs of the baby to nurse on the massage table. The massage can start in the first days for a vaginal birth, after one week for someone who had a cesarean, honoring the healing of the wound according to medical recommendations.

Many people can't afford daily massage by someone for 2-3 weeks, so doing self massage or having a friend or partner do the massage for at least some of the time is another viable option. Whoever does the massaging should remember the principles to balance Vata through massage- slow, gentle, firm, steady, integrative, repetitive massage with 4 - 8 oz of warm sesame oil. Besides calming Vata, daily massage helps the body reintegrate into its non-pregnant state. It keeps circulation going—very important for someone not moving around a lot during the recovery period. This helps prevent of the possibility of blood clots forming from blood stagnation. Massage also stimulates all the organs and energy points of the body to promote general health and emotional well being.

Warmth must be provided by keeping the room temperature comfortably warm. During and after the massage a hot water bottle can be applied to the abdomen to bring warmth deep into the Vata part of the body. Warm baths after the daily oil massage will also keep the cold of Vata from lodging in the body. This is often a favorite part of the postpartum treatment. Cold drafts should be avoided at all times.

Rest may seem illusive for a postpartum mom at times between baby care & self care. But rest she must—especially when the baby sleeps. Helpers are what can allow this to happen. If the house is a mess or other household tasks are not covered most people find it hard to rest. This is one time Ayurveda allows sleeping in the day, since the mom is recovering from childbirth and also having sleep interrupted by the baby nursing. A nap is recommended after her daily oil massage & hot bath. Sometimes soothing music can help to calm and allow rest—pick out tranquil music to use when the energy starts getting too hectic.

Many women are anxious to resume their former shape and want to exercise as soon as possible. Women should know that it is common for some to not get back to their pre-pregnancy weight for 6 months. Some women don't lose that last extra weight until they end breastfeeding and their hormones shift again. Exercise programs should not begin in earnest until after the first month and the lochia flow has ended. Doing some gentle stretches and brief walks outside later in the postpartum period will refresh and feel good without straining and using energy that would better go to the transitioning body in other ways. Deep breathing exercises, where one exhales deeply, pulling in the abdominal muscles, is a gentle way to begin toning the abdomen. Always be sure to do lots of kegel exercises postpartum to tone the pelvic floor after the work of giving birth.

Containment of the uterus by wrapping the abdomen after the massage & bath will keep Vata from staying in the space left by the baby leaving. This is a common practice in traditional cultures which proves helpful today as well. If the uterus is allowed to flop around freely while the ligaments are still loose it is more likely it will assume a position which will inhibit circulation, as well as the outflow of the lochia, causing stagnation that can lead to later problems. Arvigo Techniques of Maya Abdominal Massage® can be sure the uterus is properly positioned before applying the "faha" which holds it there if you find a properly trained and credentialed practitioner.

Quiet and seclusion are other forms of containment and important to avoid over stimulation for both mom and baby. Both are wide open and very sensitive. It's not the time for lots of out of town visitors or to have large parties of people. One case involved a baby born only 3 days earlier being brought to church and passed from person to person. Everyone was very excited & loving—but it was too much and the baby ended up getting sick.

The mom's nervous system is also reworking itself with the new levels of hormones and like the other times of hormonal change—adolescence & menopause—reducing stimulation allows for a smoother transition.

We put a sign on the door of families of newborns with a birth announcement and a "We Mother the Mother" statement requesting people who visit to stay only 15 minutes, and to lend a quick hand to do dishes, vacuum, or take a load of laundry to do. We educate the women about the importance of limiting visitors and have them warn people ahead of the birth. After the first few weeks a celebration can include everyone!

Routine & simplicity are other ways to calm Vata. When our body recognizes a rhythm happening in eating it digests better; in resting it rests better. Again, preparation ahead of birth time makes it possible to foster simplicity by being familiar with the self care routine, having meals preplanned and supported, and household needs covered.

Wholeness includes eating whole foods prepared to calm Vata, yet modified for the specific needs of postpartum women. It includes all the tastes in proportions most healthy for postpartum women, avoiding the extremes. It favors freshly harvested, seasonal and freshly cooked foods that offer clear, life giving energy, avoiding those that stress the body or add the energy of decay (such as fermented & aged foods).

Another aspect of wholeness is cultivation of the baby and mother bonding, tied closely to breastfeeding. Breastfeeding is a given in Ayurveda. If the mother avoids Vata imbalance, drinks sufficient fluids, and eats a healthy diet her milk will also be balanced. Lack of fat in the milk, too little milk is a Vata disorder. This can pass on the imbalance in her milk to the baby.

Infant massage, which can be used to encourage father and baby bonding, is another aspect of the wholeness for the baby and family. Massage is practiced universally in India and it starts as soon as the umbilical cord is healed. Then daily oil massages are given to babies before their warm bath. Randomized, controlled studies on both preterm and healthy full term infants show that massaging daily with sesame oil was most effective in promoting growth and length of time babies slept after the massage.

At the same time Vata needs attention, a postpartum woman's digestion is very often disturbed. One way to look at it is that giving birth can use every bit of energy in the body, depleting the digestive fire. It must be rekindled in the postpartum so that the food she eats is well digested to serve in making balanced milk for the baby and for her own recovery & rejuvenation. Digestive fire kindling guidelines are followed as closely as possible and digestive teas & herbs used to get things going. See Chapter "Caring for Digestion" for these guidelines.

Ayurveda and the Newborn

For the baby, leaving the contained and watery womb to go into the spacious, airy, stimulating, and relatively dry world also means a big increase in Vata dosha. So during this time Vata reduction is the basic care plan. So by keeping warm, daily oil massage & warm bath, keeping the baby's head covered with a little hat and sesame oil on the fontanelles, these all help offset Vata becoming too high in this period of time. Avoiding cold drafts is especially important.

Babies generally digest the breastmilk in about 2 hours, so constantly feeding the baby may end up depressing the digestive fire of the baby and cause digestive disturbances. Also, babies may be sensitive to some foods the mother may be eating. If the mother drinks Cumin Coriander Fennel Tea regularly it will help the baby's digestion as well as help move out any gas that may form before it becomes a tummy ache.

If the baby is having mucus problems it is often due to the mother eating too much cold food or Kapha (mucus) increasing food. However, don't cut out ALL of the Kapha foods because they are necessary for formation of the plasma which in turn forms the breast milk. Since this may be a delicate balance, take some fresh ginger tea as soon as there are signs of excess mucus beginning to show up in mother or baby. (Several cups of day would be needed in this case – otherwise use it as a general digestive once or twice a day.) As illustrated by the above examples, in general newborn babies are treated by giving the herbs to the mother.

By a couple of weeks postpartum it's possible to have a good idea of what the constitution of the baby is by how she/he looks and acts. Through this one can cultivate a suitable environment to nurture the type of personality the baby tends to have. Children in general are in the Kapha stage of life—when things are forming and are more dense. This is one reason for children having lots of mucus compared to adults.

Vata baby: Thinner, long fingers, easily distracted, when emotionally imbalanced: overwhelm
Needs a strong rhythm to lifestyle, calm, avoiding over stimulation, teaching how to be grounded.

Pitta baby: Medium, tends to be fair skinned, light thin hair or almost none, sensitive skin, wants stimulation, more focused, gets frustrated, when emotionally imbalanced: anger
Needs developmentally appropriate challenges, teaching how to relax and wind down

Kapha baby: Rounder larger, very deep "inny" belly button, calmer personality when emotionally imbalanced: clinging
Needs stimulation, teaching how to be motivated

Remember—most of us are combinations of Vata, Pitta and Kapha rather than just one pure type, so go with what seems most predominant.

By taking the advice and support of Ayurveda during the postpartum, mothers and babies will be setting the stage for a happier, longer, and healthier lives.

Snapshots of Vata-Pitta-Kapha in Postpartum

Excess Vata during Postpartum
- Sleep disturbances (especially 3 am)
- Retained lochia
- Dehydration
- Lack of appetite
- Low milk production
- After pains
- Constipation due to dryness or lack of tone

Soothing Vata during Postpartum
- Follow general Vata soothing measures as previously outlined—oiliness, internally & externally, warmth, quiet, rest
- Arvigo Techniques of Maya Abdominal Massage® recommended to be sure the uterus is placed properly. This will assist drainage. Practitioners also know about using a faha to wrap abdomen and hold the uterus in place.
- Rekindling the digestive fire-agni kindler recipe, cumin coriander & fennel tea, follow care of digestion guidelines. Eating regularly.
- Oil basti or enemas to balance the pelvic area and Vata.
- Dashmula tea- this rejuvenative for Vata downward energies and calms the pelvic area. It's recommended to drink it for four to six weeks postpartum. Dashmula is available from one of the Ayurvedic sources in the resource chapter. Boil 2 tsp of herbs in 2 cups of water, until it cooks down to ½ cup of liquid. Drink ¼ cup warm in the morning on arising. Refrigerate the rest and rewarm to drink the other ¼ cup before bed.
- Fenugreek tea- for lactation support (not for Pitta dominant women)

- Consider consulting an Ayurvedic practitioner is symptoms are not easily resolving

Excess Pitta during Postpartum
- Excessive blood loss
- Hot flashes
- Diarrhea in mother or baby

Soothing Pitta during Postpartum
- Avoid too much spice, excess heat using Pitta soothing while respecting the Vata soothing regime
- Try Pitta soothing teas (see Recipe chapter)
- Consult with an Ayurvedic practitioner in this more complicated situation

Excess Kapha during Postpartum
- Baby has mucus symptoms
- Lack of uterine involution, boggy uterus

Soothing Kapha during Postpartum
- Reduce dairy and heavy foods while respecting the Vata soothing regime
- Stimulate uterine contractions with uterine massage and appropriate herbs
- Try Kapha soothing teas (see Recipe chapter)
- Consider consulting with an Ayurvedic practitioner

Ayurvedic Recipes & Cookbooks

Herb Teas to Help Balance the Doshas

Avoiding caffeine and sugar drinks is a basic change to make for increased health. These teas are both tasty and balancing, often giving a boost in vitamins and minerals too. You can mix and match teas within a category to suit your tastebuds.

Vata Soothing Teas

- Fresh Ginger root tea—Stimulates digestion, warming and circulation, excellent for Vata. Dry ginger powder is too drying for Vata to use on a regular basis.
- Oatstraw infusions – up to one quart per day for nutritive, nerve soothing qualities
- Nettles, Red Raspberry, Red Clover infusions – up to 2 cups /day- may become too drying for Vata and in dry climates
- Vata Soothing tea – formula from Nita Desai, MD and Ayurvedic Practitioner, Boulder, CO – www.nitadesaimd.com
  - Makes 5 cups – enough for 1-2 days depending on need.
  - 1 tsp cumin seed; 1 tsp cardamom seeds; 1 tsp licorice root chunks; 1 tsp fennel seeds (these dry ingredients available from Louise Sanchez- resource listing) and 1 tsp peeled and chopped fresh ginger root. Simmer ingredients for 10 minutes, strain and drink 3-5 cups/day. Refrigerate and rewarm any left for later.

Pitta Soothing Teas

- Hibiscus tea- this is rich in iron, purifies blood, cools the pitta
- Camomile tea- digestive, balancing for Pitta
- Licorice root tea (may increase blood pressure-avoid if this is an issue) reduces heat
- Rose petal tea (be sure it's organic) -cooling, moistening, relieves inflammation
- Nettles, Red Raspberry, Red Clover, Alfalfa, Oatstraw infusions

Kapha Soothing Teas

- Licorice root tea (mildly diuretic, may increase blood pressure-avoid if this is an issue) Good for liquefying mucus so it can leave the body easier.
- Ginger powder tea -Stimulates digestion, warming, drying, and circulation, excellent for Kapha.
- Nettles, Red Raspberry, Red clover, Alfalfa infusions- up to one quart per day for nutritive, balancing qualities
- Oatstraw infusion – up to 2 cups/ day – may increase Kapha if overdone.

To make an infusion : put handful of herbs in quart jar, fill with boiling hot water, & let it sit 4-6 hours. Strain & refrigerate what you don't drink immediately. You can rewarm it as needed. Organic herbs are always the best choice.

Making Ghee

Ghee is a rejuvenative for Pitta and soothing for Vata excess. It can be used for cooking since, unlike butter, it will not burn. It is considered a very pure food and is offered in ritual fires to feed the Divine. After making this once, you are likely to do it again & again, as it is simple and not nearly so difficult as the instructions make it out to be. Homemade ghee is pure & inexpensive compared to store-bought ghee.

Preparation Time: about 30 min
   It works best to make ghee on a day that has clear skies- not cloudy

Makes about 2 cups.
-Vata, -Pitta, -Kapha

Use 1 pound organic sweet unsalted butter. Feel free to make more at a time if you want—it keeps very well
   In a heavy medium saucepan, heat butter over medium heat. Continue to cook at medium-low heat. The butter will bubble & make bubbling sounds. When it is almost done, milk solids will collect on the bottom of the pan. When it is done, in about 15 to 20 minutes, the liquid will look clear and become very quiet. Quickly take it off the heat before the milk solids on the bottom of the pan burn, which it can do suddenly (if this happens the liquid will begin to foam again rapidly and the solids turn brown instead of golden). Cool slightly. Ghee is the clear golden liquid. Pour ghee through a metal strainer &/or cheese cloth into a very clean glass. Store at room temperature. Revised from Amadea Morningstar's <u>The Ayurvedic Cookbook</u>

If you do not cook the ghee long enough, it can mold. If you cook it too long, it will let you know by burning. A touch of browning can add a nice flavor- but if it's used for ritual purposes it should not be browned.

Making Kitcheree

Kitcheree is an easily digested food that can allow the digestive system to very gently rest and cleanse. Eat only kitcheree for 1-3 days for a simple, safe cleanse that can strengthen your digestion and help break bad eating habits. Safe during pregnancy. Makes about 3 cups of kitcheree.

To make plain kitcheree:
Wash thoroughly
½ cup **split mung beans** (soak overnight to increase digestibility & reduce cooking time)**,**
1 cup **basmati rice: ,**
melt 1 Tablespoon **ghee** in a cooking pot
add **spices: 1 tsp fresh ginger, ½ tsp each tumeric, powdered cumin & coriander ;**
add rice, beans & 6 cups **water,** then bring to boil ,
turn down to simmer for <u>at least</u> 45 minutes or until mung beans are <u>very</u> soft
After cooking, add rock salt to taste. Sprinkle with chopped fresh cilantro, if desired.

You can make variations on kitcheree by adding different vegetables. See the cookbooks listed below for more ideas.

Making Agni Kindler

Agni kindler is to wake up the digestive enzymes of the stomach. Since it brings back the natural capacity is healthier for the system than relying on taking digestive enzymes. It is useful after sickness, when the appetite is low but eating is desired, or when there is a coated tongue.

For a day's supply-
Peel about 1 inch of **fresh ginger root** and grate it into fine pieces

Sprinkle with about ¼ tsp of **fresh lime juice**

Add a pinch of **unrefined salt**

Take a big pinch of this mixture 15-20 minutes before each meal.

Making Takram

Takram is drink to help digestion & absorption, taken after meals. Fresh yogurt is best used- meaning homemade yogurt. Yogurt bought in the store is usually older, making it more Pitta.

Churn 2 tablespoons of fresh yogurt in ½ cup of pure water. (The churning breaks up some of the heavy & slimy qualities of the yogurt.) Then mix in ¼ tsp cumin powder.

Making Ojas Drink - Almond Restorative Drink

This drink is important to build after a cleanse, before, during or after pregnancy to feed the ojas or underlying stamina and energy of the immune system.

Serves 1 ; V-P-K+

Soak together overnight:

10 **raw almonds** & 1 cup pure water

In the morning, drain off the water. Rub the skins off the almonds.

Bring to a boil:

1 cup **milk** (unhomogenized if possible) (milk is highly rejuvenative when digested)

Pour the milk in the blender w/ the drained & peeled almonds and :1 tablespoon organic rose petals (optional- rejuvenative), 1 tsp ghee (rejuvenative),1/32 tsp. saffron (increases digestion & rejuvenative),

1/8 tsp ground cardamom (increases diges- tion),pinch of black pepper (helps control the K),

½ tsp of sweetener (increases lactose digestion). Blend until smooth.

Drink 3-4 times/ week. Watch if any signs of excess mucous/ kapha, if so, cut back. Concentrate on increasing digestion in this case with digestive recipes taken in tandem with the ojas drink.

Making Ojas Drink - Non-dairy Versions

1. Use oat milk(if not gluten intolerant- then use almond milk) instead of cows milk. Oats are also rejuvenative, although not as strongly as cows milk.

2. Soak 20 raisins in 1 cup pure water overnight or several hours. Blend them together & use them instead of cow's milk for a rejuvenative drink. Omit sweetener in this case since the raisins are sweet enough.

Ayurvedic Cookbooks

Touching Heaven-Tonic Postpartum Recipes by Ysha Oakes – a favorite, especially designed for the postpartum

Ayurvedic Cooking for Westerners, by Amadea Morningstar – another favorite with lots of teachings

EAT•TASTE•HEAL: An Ayurvedic Cookbook for Modern Living by Thomas Yarema, MD; Daniel Rhoda; and Chef Johnny Brannigan

Ayurvedic Cooking for Self Healing By Usha Lad & Dr Vasant Lad
A virtual encyclopedia of using food for healing plus great recipes.

Resources & Reading Lists

National Ayurvedic Medicine Association
www.Ayurveda-nama.org.
Includes a list of practitioner members.

Recommended Ayurvedic Training Programs

Alandi Ashram Ayurvedic Gurukula
www.alandiashram.org
2457 20th Street, Boulder, CO 80304
303-786-7437 info@alandiashram.org

Ayurvedic Institute
www.Ayurvedicinstitute.com
P.O. Box 23445,Albuquerque, NM 87192-1445
505. 291.9698 Fax: 505.294.7572

Rocky Mtn. Institute for Yoga and Ayurveda
www.rmiya.org
P.O. Box 1091,Boulder, Colorado 80306
303.499.2910 info@rmiya.org

American Institute of Vedic Studies
www.vedanet.com
PO Box 8357, Santa Fe, NM 87504-8357
505.983.9385 vedicinst@aol.com

Sacred Window Ayurvedic Care for Mother & Baby
Ayurdoula training program
www.sacredwindow.com
12408 Hardin Ct. NE, Apt. A,
Albuquerque, NM 87111
505.508.4219

Where to Buy Ayurvedic Herbs

Banyan Botanicals, www.banyanbotanicals.com
800.952.6424 High quality herbs, most organic. Bulk herbs or encapsulated available. Pre formulated herbs available.

Ayurvedic Institute, www.Ayurvedicinstitute.com
505.291.9698 Smaller quantities of single herbs and standard mixes available.

Louise Sanchez, louise@earthnet.net
303.546.0952 Send her your formula, from this book or from an Ayurvedic practitioner (she does not do formulations for you) and she'll mix it and mail it to you. If you want it encapsulated, let her know, otherwise it's a powder.

Further Reading

Ayurveda

Ayurveda, The Science of Self-Healing by Dr Vasant Lad
This concise book covers the basics of Ayurveda, by one of the leading teachers and proponents in this country.

Ayurvedic Home Remedies by Dr. Vasant Lad
This book covers basic concepts & working with acute conditions.

Perfect Health by Deepak Chopra
This is an easy to read beginning to Ayurveda.

Ayurvedic Healing, A comprehensive guide by Dr. David Frawley

This is an in depth book with more traditional formulas and more facets of the wide field of Ayurveda.

Perfect Health for Children- Ten Ayurvedic Secrets Every Parent Should Know by Dr. John Douillard

This book by an Ayurvedic practitioner and chiropractor is written from his years of experience—and he has several children of his own, so we know it is practical.

Ayurvedic Healing for Women –Herbal Gynecology by Atreya

Offers formulas for those wishing to delve deeper into understanding using Ayurvedic herbs for gynecology.

Touching Heaven-Tonic Postpartum Care by Ysha Oakes

Ysha has shared her many years of Ayurvedic care of postpartum women in this book suitable for mothers and their caregivers. She offers a comprehensive training program at www.sacredwindow.com .

After the Baby's Birth., A Woman's Way to Wellness, by Robin Lim

Postpartum is often a neglected time for the new mother. With proper attention it can lead to great fulfillment & healing; without it this time can be exhausting & tense. This book provides perspective & resources for this time.

Preconception

Take Charge of Your Fertility by Toni Wechsler
This well written book explains the science and practicalities of fertility awareness to achieve or avoid pregnancy.

Conscious Conception, by Jeanine Parvati Baker
Full of amazing information and tales about conscious conception around the world, written by one of my favorite wisewomen.

The Whole Person Fertility Program, by Niravi Payne
Addresses emotional issues that may interfere with fertility--- and healthy pregnancy, birth & mothering.

Pregnancy & Childbirth

Active Birth, by Janet Balaskas
Most closely mirrors my own homebirth practice. It includes exercises to prepare for birthing, great pictures, and a chapter on water birth.

Special Delivery, by Rahima Baldwin
Explains pregnancy & birth from a natural perspective which is useful for homebirth or any other place one wishes to have a natural experience.

Pregnant Feelings, Developing Trust in Birth, by Rahima Baldwin Dancy & Terra Palmarini Richardson (Now known as Terra Rafael)
Focuses on the emotional aspects of the childbearing year, with a workbook format. Helpful for getting perspective on fears, beliefs, & other emotions that come to the

surface so easily at this time of transition. Available used on line—currently out of print.

The Birth Partner, by Penny Simkin, PT
Excellent for those interested in a hospital birth. It gives information about birth & about what to expect in the hospital, what kinds of decisions you may need to make about care, and alternatives to use from least interventive to highly interventive, according to needs.

Birthing From Within by Pam England & Rob Horowitz
Another popular book to work with emotional preparation for labor.

Wisewoman Herbal for the Childbearing Year, by Susun Weed
Very helpful if you would like to use herbal & other natural helps at this time in your life.

Focus on the Child

The Magical Child, by Joseph Chilton Pearce
Explains the importance of the mother-child bond immediately after birth as the basis for further development and goes on through childhood. Compelling.

The Amazing Newborn, by Klaus & Kennel
With great photos, this book illustrates just how intelligent and aware newborn babies are.

Breastfeeding Your Baby, by Sheila Kitzinger
Any book by Sheila is great - this one focuses on the breastfeeding experience, with lots of good pictures & experiences of mothers.

Our Babies, Ourselves by Meredith F. Small

Based on research, Meredith explores why we parent the way we do and how to become more aware in our choices. I couldn't put it down.

Your Baby & Child, by Penelope Leach

Complete book on child development. It is mainstream, yet not very dogmatic. I have turned to it time & again for assurance - reading that others go through similar stages & problems is helpful to keep perspective.

Smart Medicine for a Healthier Child, by Zand, Walton & Rountree

These authors are Colorado practitioners who are well versed in using nutritional supplements, herbs, homeopathy, acupressure, diet & conventional medicine to suit the situation. A good reference to work with.

Midwifery

Holistic Midwifery Vol I & II by Anne Frye
Excellent text for midwifery.

Spiritual Midwifery by Ina May Gaskin
Filled with stories from the early days of the American homebirth resurgence

About the Author

Terra Rafael is a **Registered Midwife** and attended births for over 20 years, while teaching over 150 midwifery students & apprenticing several in her practice. She became a Reiki Master in June, 1999 and graduated from Alandi Ayurvedic School as an **Ayurvedic Practitioner** in May 2001. Terra completed certification as a practitioner in the **Arvigo Techniques of Maya Abdominal Massage®**, having begun her maya massage work Fall, 2002, while completing an apprenticeship to Miss Beatrice Waight, maya midwife & shamanic healer from Belize in March, 2003.

She is now **writing** and publishing her works. Previous books include:
Pregnant Feelings, Developing Trust in Birth, coauthored with Rahima Baldwin Dancy
Giving Birth to Ourselves, contemplations for midwives
Work in **A Week's Worth of Women**, edited by Jyoti Wind

Watch for her upcoming titles:
Remembering the Art of Midwifery – Journey to the Great Midwife
Reunion with Mother Nature – essays and memoir

Terra continues her **healing work with women** through her practice **WiseWomanhood**.
See more about Terra and her work at:
www.womanways.blogspot.com
www.aweeksworthofwomen.blogspot.com (on Mondays)
www.facebook.com/WiseWomanhood

Contact Terra at:
wisewomanhood@gmail.com